MIRACLE
at Exit Number 3

MIRACLE
at Exit Number 3

THOMAS KELLY COOPER

TATE PUBLISHING
AND ENTERPRISES, LLC

Published by Tate Publishing & Enterprises, LLC
127 E. Trade Center Terrace | Mustang, Oklahoma 73064 USA
1.888.361.9473 | www.tatepublishing.com

Tate Publishing is committed to excellence in the publishing industry. The company reflects the philosophy established by the founders, based on Psalm 68:11,
"The Lord gave the word and great was the company of those who published it."

Cover design by Jan Sunday Quilaquil
Interior design by Joana Quilantnga

Published in the United States of America

ISBN: 978-1-63063-929-7
Biography & Autobiography / General
14.02.05

DEDICATION

This book is dedicated to my wife, Karen, and to my daughters, Kelly and Jennifer, and to their future families. It is dedicated to Ed who provided the gift that allowed me to experience life with my wife, daughters, family, and friends. It is dedicated to my sister Mildred and my brother Billy whose constant and unwavering support and encouragement has helped me to persevere through the storms and joys of life.

Of course, the book must be dedicated to our parents who gave to us the most precious gift of all—a fighting chance at life. Their love and devotion has been a gift far beyond what they could have imagined or expected. It is dedicated to Gayle, Rusty, and Laurie whose courage, love, and friendship are unwavering.

It is dedicated to all of my nieces and nephews and to all of our family at the cabin and beyond. It is dedicated to Elaine and Jeannie who were friends before I married their little sister. It is dedicated to each of their spouses, children, and grandchildren.

It is dedicated to all who have donated or will someday donate the gift of life and to all who have received the gift of life from others. Most people will never be confronted with the choice of whether or not to donate life. If you are, my prayer is that regardless of your decision, other lives will be strengthened and enhanced by your actions. My prayer is that this book would be an encouragement to individuals and families to stay strong and keep the faith.

ACKNOWLEDGMENTS

It is with much gratitude that I thank my sister Mildred for her wonderful contributions that have helped to make this book possible. She has given her time and encouragement in addition to the many hours spent reading and editing the narrative. She along with brothers Billy and Ed have shared their memories of our parents and grandparents as well as many events of our childhood. Without their input, this book would have been much more difficult.

My part of the story, for the last thirty-five years, would not have been possible without the gift of life that Ed gave to me so many years ago. Thirty-five years is the equivalent of 12,785 days, each of which, though sometimes difficult, has been a blessing.

My wife, Karen, has provided invaluable support. With great patience, she has read the narrative and provided inspiration. She has helped guide me when I was unsure and helped me stay focused and on topic.

I give thanks to God who has been with me on each and every step of this journey on earth. Discovering the mercy and loving kindness that he has for each and all of his creation has been one of the great pleasures of life. I stand amazed at the way things seem to have worked themselves out. Life is an amazing gift from God.

Many friends, both old and new, have encouraged me to write this story. I deeply appreciate each of you and the kind words you have expressed toward me and my family. I hope the finished work may somehow be worthy of your expectations.

My parents, Bill and June, deserve so much of the acknowledgment for this story. They taught their children by their own example and gave each of us the opportunity to find our way and to begin our own journey down life's pathway.

CONTENTS

We are not all called to run the same race; we each have our own race to run. As a result of us running our race successfully, by the grace of God and for his glory, we inspire others to run their race with the same intentional purpose. It is not equal sacrifice but equal servitude. As we each serve God faithfully in the capacity he has called us, we inspire others and build the body of Christ up in love.

PROLOGUE

MAMA'S YELLOW BUTTERFLY

Mildred Cooper Russell

Mildred has lived in Florida with her family for a number of years. She shares the following story about her last visit with our mom and mama's yellow butterfly.

It was a special time, the month that my mother spent with us that last year of her life. I was having an operation on my foot, and I asked her to come down and be with me. It was an excuse to get her here; I didn't really want her to do anything much but be here with me and my family. We cherished our time with her, and we had so little of it. She agreed to stay for the month of February. I was ecstatic!

When Mother arrived, we were shocked at her condition. Her legs were horribly swollen, her lips were blue, and she was short of breath. I urged her to go to a heart specialist here—our town has a hospital noted for its cardiac care. She did not want to, and no amount of coaxing could persuade her. Seeing that she would not change her mind, I decided to concentrate on doing the things we enjoyed and making her visit as pleasant as possible.

One day when we were in the backyard looking at our plants, she saw a yellow butterfly. "Oh, there is my yellow butterfly," she said. "I wondered where he went in the winter. I'm glad he comes here to stay with you. He stays with me in the summer." We laughed at the thought of a butterfly visiting back and forth summer and winter, but that comment has meant a lot to me in the years since her death.

On many occasions, I have seen a yellow butterfly and thought of Mother. The day that my daughter Rebekah conquered her fear of the ocean, I saw a yellow butterfly at the beach of all places and thought of Mother. She would have loved to see her granddaughter splashing gleefully in the waves. It may seem silly to some, but I thought that it may have been God's way of letting me know that somehow my mother was still sharing our joys.

When my youngest brother and his family visited one summer, we went tubing on the Itchetuckne River. As we floated down the river enjoying the calm of the day and our beautiful surroundings, I saw a yellow butterfly. I saw it again as we rode the tram back to the starting point. I told my brother about the butterfly, and he too understood the significance of it. Mother never did float down the river with us, but her butterfly has gone with us every time since that first day I saw him.

On many other occasions, not special in themselves, I have seen a yellow butterfly and have always thought of my mother. Whenever I am doing something with my family, or alone, and I see a yellow butterfly, the event becomes more meaningful. Seeing the butterfly seems somehow to be a seal of approval, almost as good as a smile from Mother would have been.

Many things my brothers and our children say and do remind me of Mother, and I know she lives on in us. Sometimes I find myself wondering if Mother would think the same thing I do about a book I read or a movie I saw. I want to tell her about the things the children do that make us so proud and share the heartaches that their growing up can bring. I am happy to say that her yellow butterfly has stayed with me year round, and it is a sweet reminder that she loved me, and my family, and that we had a very special visit, which left me with a unique way to remember that love.

CELEBRATING LIFE

When Ed and I walked into the conference room at the Vanderbilt University Transplant Center, we were instantly transported back in time. Ms. Jane was the first to greet us, and Jeannie was right next to her. We were all quite a bit older, but the connection of spirit had not waned. Ms. Jane was always there to check us into the clinic and make sure we did what we were supposed to do. Jeannie was the transplant coordinator who made everything else work. How wonderful it was to see them again and give them a hug.

Dr. Ritchie, one of the transplant surgeons, was there, having made the trip from Florida where he has been enjoying retirement for several years. I met with Dr. H. Keith Johnson, who is the transplant nephrologists for Ed and me, at a clinic visit prior to the luncheon. It was the first time I had seen him in many years.

It was a very special privilege to meet several of the doctors, coordinators, nurses, and staff members of the current transplant program. Our surgeries, in February of 1979, were done in the old Vanderbilt Hospital, which is the same place where I had major life-saving surgery at twenty-one months of age.

That lung surgery took the lower lobe of my right lung. The complications that followed foreshadowed years of health concerns about chronic lung disease. A new magnificent Vanderbilt University Medical Center complex was completed just a few years after the kidney transplant.

I remember my mom telling people how wonderful the nurses, doctors, and support staff at Vanderbilt had been to her during the traumatic events in 1955. The doctors and staff at Vanderbilt are still among the best in the world, and the quality of care is as impressive today as it was back in the day.

At the time of the reception, it had been thirty years since Ed donated the gift of life to me, in the form of his right kidney. The resulting transplant ended eighteen months of dialysis for me and saved my life. We were at a luncheon to honor Ed and all of those who were a part of that event so many years ago. We cannot forget the hope our parents had that day tempered by the concern for two sons going into surgery.

We could not thank everyone who had been a part of the transplant experience at this luncheon because most were not there. Almost everyone involved had retired and moved on. It was difficult to locate and invite many of the participants. And how do you say thanks for more than three decades of life?

Dr. Jackson, an internal medicine physician in Paducah, Kentucky, where we lived at the time of the transplant, who guided me through dialysis and then onto transplant, had died several years earlier. He had suffered from a very painful condition since birth and was as much a role model to me as he was a physician.

The staff at Lourdes Hospital in Paducah is also due many thanks. Special thanks go to the dialysis staff in what was the new dialysis unit in the basement of the hospital. The hemodialysis unit first opened in May 1973 with only one machine. In 1977, when I first started dialysis, there were six kidney machines in operation and one backup unit.

The unit received patients from more than a one-hundred-mile radius of the Paducah area. The travel time from my house to undergo the four-hour, three-times-a-week treatment was approximately ten minutes. Louisville or Nashville was the primary choice for dialysis before Lourdes began the regional services program, and they were both several hours away.

The dedicated teams of medical professionals deserve our continued thanks. Nurses, transplant coordinators, nephrologists, urologists, anesthesiologists, pulmonologists, social workers, and all others involved in the field of transplantation, then and now, worked tirelessly in sometimes tragic situations to help restore the health of each patient.

And this was really a celebration for the many thousands who have donated or received the gift of life before and since that day and, hopefully, encouragement and inspiration for the countless numbers that today wait for a life-saving transplant, including hundreds of children.

I recently opened the old, dented black trunk that my mom gave me when I went away to college and once again looked at the dozens of "get well" cards and letters that were sent our way before and after the surgery. I saved them all. They still serve as a reminder to me of the positive impact that simple acts of love and friendship directed toward a person can have on that individual.

We could not have known back then that we would one day become Vanderbilt's longest surviving transplant donor and recipient or one of the longest surviving pair of brother-to-brother organ donor and recipient in the world. We would much rather acknowledge the donors and the many thousands of successful transplants that have occurred since. Life is so very precious, and tomorrow is promised to no one.

My brother chose to donate life back in the days of the wild wild west of organ transplants, as one doctor recently described it. Ed was a pioneer and a trailblazer in the field of organ donation and transplant and remains an inspiration to all who know his story. His life has been one that has made his family and friends proud for many reasons, not the least of which is his decision to donate life or him becoming one of the longest surviving organ donors in the world.

Laurie, Ed's girlfriend, and later his wife, visited Ed in the hospital after the surgery. I sometimes kid Ed about the fact that after the surgery, he refused to take any pain medication because he wanted to be strong for his girlfriend. Most people will agree that the pain after surgery is greater for the donor than the recipient. But I know that he refused the medication because that is just the way he is—always meeting challenges head on and then anticipating the next one.

Ed was working part-time at Paducah Drug Company while attending his second semester of college. He would miss several weeks of work because of the surgery, but when he returned, it was his time to receive a special gift. The owners of the company paid him his regular wage for the average hours he would have worked had he not donated life, a gift he would never forget.

He did not return to class that semester, but all of his teachers were very supportive and accommodating. They prepared and sent him lesson plans so that he could keep up with the class material. Some of the students made copies of their class notes and gave them to him. Ed made all As that semester.

Many of the teachers knew our mom and dad and had also been my teacher when I attended the college a few years earlier. And a few of the students knew both Ed and me. One of the students asked a fellow student if she knew that Ed was about to donate one of his kidneys to his brother. She did know that. And as life goes, the young lady to whom the question was addressed would become my wife in a little less than five years.

On the morning of the surgery, Mrs. Price's 8:00 a.m. English literature class paused to offer prayers for us and our family. A few days earlier, Concord United Methodist Church, where my parents were charter members and where our family had worshipped for years, had asked Ed and me to attend a special prayer service. We were asked to come to the front where the pastor and congregation joined around us in a circle and asked God for a safe and successful transplant. Other churches across the country, as a congregation and as individual members, had prayed for us as well.

We did not think that much about longevity as the years passed. There was work to be done along with marriage and raising a family. We each have traveled extensively around the country, and we, like many donors and recipients, have volunteered time, when we could, and have shared our story to various audiences to raise awareness and assist in the effort to save lives through organ donation.

Family was at the reception too. Our brother Bill, the oldest of three brothers; his wife, Gayle; their daughter, Karen; and her family had made the hour long trip from Tullahoma, Tennessee, to celebrate the milestone. Ed's oldest daughter, Katie, and her husband, Tie, also attended the reception. Mildred, our only sister; her husband, Henry; and their children were unable to attend.

It has been more than thirty-four years now since transplant day. On the upcoming thirty-fifth anniversary of transplant day, 12,785 days will have passed since Ed donated the gift of life. That's the equivalent of 1,826 weeks plus 2 days or 306,816 hours. It has not always been easy for either one of us, but each minute of the thirty-five years has been a blessing.

Despite being one of the world's longest surviving organ donors, Ed has never had any issues arise from his decision to donate. His health remains good and he has never had any problem obtaining health insurance as a result of the living donation. He continues to reassure anyone who may ask that he has never had any regrets about his decision.

This book is, in part, a tribute to Ed for his decision to donate the gift of life more than thirty-five years ago. His gift has continued to give over the years allowing the recipient to live a long and productive life. He is an everyday hero and a great example of someone who lay down his life to save someone else.

He remains a very humble man about his experience, insisting that he is not a hero. He believes that he did what he had to do and never considered any other options. Everyone who donates is a hero to someone. And, though there are no guarantees, there is a very real possibility that their gift will continue to give for a lifetime.

He hopes that people would consider living organ donation, as well as donation after death, and perhaps, in some way, benefit from his experience. Ed says that being a living donor has not caused him to make any significant changes in his lifestyle. He has continued to be active in sports, stays in shape, and controls his weight as all of us would need to do. And, he enjoys food and beverages in moderation.

Our story has been difficult to write for a number of reasons. It is about so much more than Ed and me and our journey together, the transplant, or the time that has since passed. This is a story for all families and people who have struggled with the many difficult circumstances of life over the years. It is the story of unconditional love and the discovery of what makes life such a gift.

The gift of life is enhanced, and indeed made possible, by the many painful decisions that our parents made and the courage they had and in turn poured into their children. It is also the story of how faith in God, trust in people, and forgiveness play such a vital and dramatic role in the healing process of the human body.

My brothers and sister and I have always been close. We often think alike, but we seem to occasionally arrive at the conclusions from somewhat different perspectives. We have shared many of the joys and sorrows of life together and individually. We can sometimes sense each other's thoughts and often communicate without speaking. There is an unbreakable bond of love and common inheritance, though we have each traveled different, yet similar paths.

Perhaps this can be explained, in part, by the difference in age. Billy was almost nineteen and away at college when Ed was born. Mildred is seven years younger than Billy and four years older than I. I am seven years older than Ed.

Billy had graduated from the University of Mississippi and was in the navy during the Vietnam War when Ed was starting first grade. Yet we all attended the same elementary school, middle school, and high school. We each had some of the same high school teachers.

Billy was voted the most likely to succeed by his senior classmates at Heath High School. That was a particularly tough act to follow as Mildred, then me, and then Ed would each follow him and graduate from the same high school. The four of us had several of the same teachers over that twenty-two-year period.

Billy and Mildred, for a season, shared a home and church when the family lived in our father's hometown of Purvis, Mississippi. Ed and I would be born later, in Kentucky, and never lived in Mississippi. They lived near relatives and grandparents when very young. Ed and I never had relatives living close at hand.

However, we all lived in the same house in Paducah, Kentucky, and enjoyed the land around it. Billy lived there for thirteen years before entering the navy. Mildred lived there for seventeen years while I was there eighteen and Ed eleven.

The four of us tell four different stories completely intertwined over our entire lifetimes. When each of the stories joins together, they chronicle one family's struggles and accomplishments over the many years. They are stories of tragedy and triumph and of humor and sorrow.

The following is an article written after the reception at Vanderbilt observing the thirtieth anniversary of the transplant. It was published in the House Organ, a publication of Vanderbilt University Medical Center, in the June 2009 issue.

> To save a brother
>
> How do you say thanks
> for three decades of life?
>
> By Jessica Pasley
>
> Growing up, Ed Cooper always looked up to his older brother, Tom. So it was quite fitting for him to be the one to save his brother's life.
>
> "He was seven years older than I was," said Ed. "He's the one who helped me learn to read and write, throw a baseball, hit a baseball. He has always been my hero.
>
> When the doctors said that he would definitely need a transplant, I told my parents that I was ready to be tested. There was not much to think over.
>
> "I really don't consider it anything special on my part because I think most people in that situation and with that opportunity would do the same thing."

It's been 30 years since Ed, 49, donated his kidney to his older brother Tom, 56.

Recently the brothers, Vanderbilt's longest surviving living donor and recipient, returned to Vanderbilt to observe the anniversary. A reception was held in their honor. The pair was able to visit with some old friends who have since retired from the Vanderbilt Transplant Center.

In 1999, 20 years post transplant, Tom was the second longest living kidney recipient at Vanderbilt. According to 2008, data there are 70 living donor patients worldwide surviving for 30 years or more, with 49 of those survivors living in the United States. Vanderbilt's first living donor transplant was performed in 1970.

The milestone is one the brothers have been only too happy to celebrate, because in 1967 a kidney failure diagnosis was considered a death sentence.

No hesitation

When Tom was 9 months old, doctors discovered that his kidneys were damaged from crystallized sulfur drugs. At 14, the family was told that Tom's kidneys would probably fail in about 10 years.

Over the years, his kidneys slowly deteriorated, but it did not keep him from a normal childhood. It wasn't until he was 24 that his health status began to change. Although dialysis became routine, it was evident that the regime was no longer useful.

"I didn't really feel bad," said Tom. "I didn't really know what feeling good was, but I felt as good as far as I knew. I had been pretty active in school and in sports. But once I graduated from college and started my first job, things began to change."

Ed was tested and found to be a perfect match. "Ed never hesitated," said Tom. "It was quite encouraging to me. My life has been amazing. I have been very blessed and fortunate to have my faith and my family because they have brought me through a lot.

"Because of what Ed did, I have been able to have a normal life. I understand that it is a special gift and that not everyone has this opportunity, but by his giving me one of his kidneys I was able to live."

Tom, retired from the Federal Bureau of Prisons, lives in Fredericksburg, Virginia with his wife, Karen. They've been married 25 years and have two daughters.

Ed was a freshman in college when the donation process began. During the examination period, doctors discovered that Ed's left kidney had three arteries, while his right kidney had two. Typically, a kidney has a single artery and traditionally the medical team removes the donor's left kidney for transplantation. This raised the stakes for Ed's role as a donor and the transplant was postponed.

But six months later Ed got the call that would save his brother's life.

"I was at work," said Ed. "They came over the PA system and said I had a call from someone with the Vanderbilt transplant team. I remember them saying, 'We decided to take the right kidney and make it work if you are willing to think about it.'"

"I remember saying 'what was there to think about?' We need to do it. That was a defining moment for me and knowing that it was all going to really happen.

Great testimony

Both brothers woke up surrounded by their parents, Bill and June, who are now deceased. Ed was allowed to leave the hospital 10 days after the surgery, while Tom stayed 21 days, and both have been healthy since.

"Physically I have never had any limitation or problems," said Ed. "Even though I am involved with Tennessee Donor Services, I don't want any attention for what I did. One of the most rewarding parts of all of this is being able to tell his story in hopes that it will bring awareness to others."

Ed, who lives in Nashville, has been married 28 years and has two daughters and a son. His personal experience propels him before others in an effort to raise awareness. But having a family has been an eye opening experience as well.

During his many talks and volunteer opportunities, Ed admits that if he can help educate one person, the good it can do is far reaching.

"Oftentimes, people have to have a personal experience with organ donation to understand the crisis and shortage or even how easy it is to sign up. But if you can enlighten that one person, who can share with someone else, the gift continues.

"People who receive transplanted organs, and those who are able to be living donors, often have very full and healthy lives. That in itself is a great testimony."

ONE MISSISSIPPI—DEEP ROOTS

It was sad that our mom and dad could not be at the thirty-year transplant reception at Vanderbilt since they are such a significant part of this story. This story could not be understood except in the context of our entire family and the sacrifices and contributions they too made. We will always remember their unwavering support and encouragement. And we will never forget the concern on our parents' faces as they watched two sons taken to surgery.

Our mother would sometimes tell us that the sun shines and the rain falls on everyone. That was not usually what we wanted to hear at a moment when we were sick or discouraged, feeling like the only person in the world whom God had forgotten and wondering why this had happened to me. But if anyone would know for sure, it would me our mom.

We would learn from her, and then from experience, that everyone faces unique challenges in life. The most important thing is how you respond to them. Our dad was not much help either. More often than not, when we would ask him for help at a particular task, he would get that special look on his face, a quizzical yet serious "marine corps" look, and ask us if we were capable of figuring it out for ourselves. Usually, after getting the answer to that question wrong a few times, we would indeed accomplish our mission, or he would relent and offer some supportive advice that would help us complete the task.

They would be there for us, their four children, during good times and bad, during the early years of our lives. We would watch as their faith was tested over and over again and then stand amazed as they, with faith validated, pushed forward, overcoming the challenges while instinctively, though unconsciously, teaching us to never give up.

Our parents were not unaccustomed to the devastating effects of physical pain. Our dad suffered an injury while serving in the Marine Corps in Haiti. Most of the veins in his left leg were stripped out. Though not constant, he would, at times, bear the resulting pain and discomfort for the rest of his life. He would become a member of the Disabled American Veterans. He also contracted dinghy fever and suffered a ruptured appendix while in Haiti.

Our mom sustained a back injury when she was young that would cause intense pain on occasion. She had surgery on two separate occasions after Ed was born. The surgeries helped but did not alleviate periodic episodes of intense pain. They rarely complained about their circumstances, and even those closest to them were often unaware of the pain they were enduring when the episodes recurred.

They survived the great depression and World War II and then built a successful business starting with nothing but their hopes of a better future. As a young married couple, our parents experienced the enormous challenges of a child's illness when their firstborn child suffered from polio. Their second child, and only daughter, struggled at times with severe asthma. Like many families, they faced painful decisions and did what they had to do. For our family, like all families, there were many unexpected twists and turns, heartbreak, and joy.

Perhaps the greatest common gifts, we, their children, each have, are our parents and the legacy they handed down to us. June Elaine Waggoner was born in Carthage, Mississippi. She was the youngest of nine children, seven of whom survived through infancy.

Her father was elected to the position of superintendent of schools, in Carthage, and was serving his second term when he died suddenly leaving June, nine years old at the time, her mom, and brothers alone in the middle of the Great Depression. His wife, Belle, won the special election to replace him and finished his term as superintendent. She then lost the subsequent election to serve for a full term. One other woman was elected to office in Leake County at the same time as our grandmother. They were the first two women to be elected to office in the county.

Times were hard for almost everyone, and when her husband died and her reelection bid failed, she also lost her primary source of income. They lived a few more years in Carthage, and then Mamma Belle and June moved to Washington, DC, for a time to live with one of June's brothers and his family. This move was after June's junior year of high school, and she would graduate, after completing her senior year in Washington.

It was quite a culture shock for the young June to suddenly be living in the nation's capital so far from the security of the small town and farm where she had grown up surrounded by family and friends. But as was her nature, with an adventurous spirit, she adjusted quickly, making friends and learning the customs, sights, sounds, and rules of city life. She joined a women's basketball team and took swimming lessons at the YWCA.

Though she would never live in Carthage again, we would visit there often over the years. We would visit for the yearly family reunions often held on the grounds of Bethel Methodist Church, the old family church at Rocky Hill, or for funerals in the family cemetery next to Bethel church. We would retrace the steps of her childhood and listen to the stories of her youth.

Unwittingly, it seems, and over time, we would begin to piece together the fabric of her life's journeys and begin to better understand the events that shaped such a passionate and curious soul. In doing so, it seems we may somewhat better understand ourselves.

She lived in a place where Choctaw Indian children played alongside black and white children. She lost a classmate who drowned in the river during a school outing. The trees, rocks, flowers, and streams each seemed to tell a special story that she carefully listened to and learned to understand. Her love of nature and its surrounds were a treasure that she would pass onto each of us.

It was in Washington that she met William Burt Cooper, an acquaintance of her brother. Bill was from Purvis, Mississippi, and the common heritage must have certainly played a role in the attraction. Bill was a former marine marksman and sharpshooter who served four years in the corps, part of the time with the marines in Haiti. He was on the last boat of American service men to leave the island when the United States pulled out of Haiti in 1934. When his service was finished, he moved to Washington where he attended college and worked.

The Waggoners and Coopers have a long history of military service going at least as far back as the American Revolution. And few families spilled more blood on behalf of the Confederacy than the Waggoners of Leake County. They sent six sons to war. Four of them were killed. A fifth was taken prisoner twice but survived to return with the youngest brother, who served as a youth of sixteen. Vess was with Lee's army at the surrender site at Appomattox Court House.

The youngest brother, William Cicero Waggoner, is June's grandfather. Henry and Martha Waggoner, parents of the brave men, moved to Madison County, Mississippi, from Georgia in 1845 and then to Leake County in 1852.

The Waggoners came by their valor naturally. Their grandfather and at least one uncle had seen service from Georgia in the American Revolution. This is a source of family pride; we are American back to and before the revolution. June would become a member of the Daughters of the American Revolution (DAR).

Our father's grandfather also served during the American Civil War. He was eventually captured at the battle of Nashville and was taken to Camp Douglas, the infamous prisoner of war camp in Chicago, Illinois. That family had three sons killed in the war.

Bill and June were married the October after her high school graduation in 1939. William Burt Cooper Jr. was born in 1941. In December of 1941, the Japanese attacked Pearl Harbor, and America was once again at war.

Our parents and Billy moved from Washington, DC, during the early months of World War II, to Purvis, Mississippi, our dad's hometown. Billy was about eighteen months old when they were in Purvis the first time. Daddy helped install the steam heat in the buildings at Camp Shelby, near Purvis, during World War II. He also worked for a time in Gulfport, Mississippi.

It was during this first time in Purvis when Billy first met Georgia Mae Robinson. She was about five years older than mother and already had two daughters. She was married to R. C. Robinson and had grown up near York, Alabama. Mother and daddy were looking for someone to help with Billy. He remembers, "When Georgia Mae came, they talked to her and decided that if I would go to her, she could have the job. It was an instant bond. And of course, Georgia Mae has been a part of the life of our family ever since."

Mildred, our only sister, talks about her memories of Georgia Mae. "A special treat this trip was a visit with the lady I can only affectionately think of as my nanny. She was in fact a friend to our family, who did work for us but did far more. She stayed with us when my brother had polio and we were quarantined. She loved us and spoiled us.

"She came to Kentucky when Tom was born and then when he had to have emergency surgery. I vaguely remember thinking that she was part of our family and did not understand why she did not go with us to Kentucky. I know she has much to tell me that I have forgotten or never knew. I hope to go back one day soon and spend several hours with her. She brings the same joy to my heart now that she did when I was a small child, loved and fussed over by everyone I knew."

After Purvis, the family moved to Oak Ridge, Tennessee, where a top secret government facility was being built. This would later be known as the Manhattan Project. Daddy was a steam fitter and pipe fitter working at this gaseous diffusion plant that produced the material for the first atomic bomb.

People working on the Manhattan Project were not allowed to leave base and were told to never discuss what their job duties were during this time. Daddy would tell us of friends he would meet decades later that had also worked on the project and still would not discuss their duties. They never forgot that "loose lips sink ships."

Billy's earliest memories were from Oak Ridge when he was three years old. He remembers, "We lived in K-25, a very large area of two-room trailers. The front room was a living room, dining room, kitchen, and the second room was a bedroom. I slept in the back room. Mother and Daddy slept on a couch in the front room."

When the job was finished at Oak Ridge, and on the day after Billy's fourth birthday, the family packed up and headed toward Baton Rouge, Louisiana, where another job was waiting. Billy remembered the day they left Oak Ridge for Louisiana. "We left Oak Ridge late in the afternoon in a one-seat Plymouth Coupe with a large shelf behind the seat. They made a bed for me on the shelf. We pulled a small trailer. It was similar to a U-Haul all-metal trailer.

That first afternoon as it was getting dark, we were heading down a mountain when Daddy made the comment, 'A wheel just passed us. Someone behind us has lost a wheel.' About that time, he discovered it was a wheel from our trailer. A friendly soul chased it and brought it back. Most folks did things like that then. They all knew that someday they would be the one needing the assistance."

The family lived in Baton Rouge for a short period before moving back to Purvis where Daddy had purchased a farm. Billy was now about five years old, and they hoped that this would be the last move home. Those days were some of Billy's fondest memories, and he told us about the farm.

"The farm consisted of 160 acres. It was about ten minutes from town. The nearest neighbor, the Johnson family, lived toward town almost a mile away. Boggy Hollow Creek was down the hill from our house about a quarter of a mile. The creek was spring fed. It came out of the swamp and saw the light of day for the first time at the bridge across our road. The water at that spot was very cold! On the hottest day of the summer, you could spend five minutes in the water and have blue lips for hours."

It was open-range country, which meant there were no fences to keep the neighbors livestock separated. It was one of the great pleasures of life to listen as they tell the stories of those treasured memories of days before my sister and me and my younger brother were born.

Mildred Elaine Cooper was born in Purvis during this time and recalled what she had been told. Mother had insisted on moving into town because there was no phone or electricity at the farm. "My older brother was seven when I was born. I am told that he prayed for a little sister, though when I was a toddler and was tearing his room apart, he regretted the answer for a little while. My parents were glad to have a girl.

The doctor said to my mother, 'Thank goodness it's a girl.' She hadn't realized that it was so obvious that she would like a girl to go with her boy. I was the first baby that my doctor delivered after he finished residency and went into private practice. So many blessings surrounded me in my early days, so much love. I will always be thankful for that place where I had my beginnings and the people who were there to welcome me.

"Our grandparents, my father's parents, were another special link to my early days. My grandfather had been the county sheriff. He worked at the post office when I was born. I am told that a highlight of my day was going to visit my papaw. He was a quiet and gentle man. He took me for a ride around the block in his car every night. I could not go to sleep until this evening ritual was performed. I would miss this most of all when we moved far away to Kentucky. Being too young to understand how far away we were, I was miserable for a long time because I missed my grandfather so much."

In addition to farming, Daddy owned and operated a hardware store in Purvis. Billy became a familiar figure around town. After catching a ride or walking to town, he could often be seen selling popcorn or engaging neighbors on the street near the county courthouse, hardware store, or post office.

The hardware store business did well for a while, but eventually, hard economic times forced Daddy to close it down. Another job was waiting in Kentucky. Mother was not certain about the move and asked God to give her a sign. The radio was on in the hardware store, and right after Mother prayed, "My Old Kentucky Home" began playing on the radio. She took that as a yes to the move.

So our parents, with Billy and Mildred, moved from the beloved hometown of Purvis to McCracken County, near Paducah, Kentucky. Billy recalls the travel to Paducah. "Mother, Mildred, and I left Purvis August 11, 1951. Papaw took us to Hattiesburg where we got on a bus headed to Jackson, Mississippi. At Jackson, we boarded a passenger train, the now famous *The City of New Orleans*, northbound to Fulton, Kentucky. Fulton was the closest passenger rail station to Paducah at the time.

Daddy met the train, which was about an hour and a half late, and we headed to Paducah. We ate supper at Mrs. Perry's boarding house where daddy had been staying." Daddy worked at the Shawnee coal fired steam generating plant which would produce electricity for the gaseous diffusion plant which produced enriched, weapon grade uranium.

And this would be the place where the story of exit number 3 would one day begin to unfold. Our parents had met the challenges and persevered though childhoods of modest means, the Great Depression, World War II, painful injuries, and the illnesses of their oldest child. With unwavering faith in God, they would now embark on another journey, which would bring new but yet unknown accomplishment, joy, and heartache.

Perhaps the miracle is that, thanks to God, they had come this far. But more of the miraculous in the midst of great testing lay ahead. The first exit off the newly built interstate highway, heading south after crossing the Ohio River from Illinois into Kentucky, a doorway to Dixie, would one day be designated as exit number 3.

GHOSTS OF EXIT 3

Our parents purchased a house and farm sitting on forty-seven acres when they moved to Paducah, Kentucky. Ed and I were both born in Paducah. My parents endured the loss of a baby girl in 1956 when my mom suffered a miscarriage. Following this tragic loss, my parents decided that the family was complete and that they would not have more children.

A new medical procedure, called a vasectomy, had just become available, and our dad had completed the procedure shortly after the miscarriage. Nevertheless, amazingly, and thankfully, God blessed our world a couple of years later with the birth of their youngest child, Edward Andrew.

The house into which the family moved when they arrived in Paducah had coal oil heat and no air conditioning. We had well water to drink. The water was pure and the well never ran dry unless Mother forgot to turn off the hose while watering her beautiful roses or other flowers. Running the well dry was a source of irritation for Daddy, one of the few I can recall. There was a heavy metal top with a handle over the well. We were not supposed to take the cover off, and we rarely got to look down into the well. Occasionally, the pump would need to be primed, and Mama or Daddy would go out and remove the cover and restart the pump.

Later on, the kitchen would be enlarged and remodeled, and a small family room would be added. Central heat and air were installed, and city water eventually arrived. An office for my dad's growing accounting business was built adjoining the house.

Roughly fifteen tall majestic old oak trees graced one side of the front yard from the house out to the road. Over time, the number or trees slowly decreased, mostly as a result of lightning or tornado winds.

This was not the piney woods and open range down by the muddy Pearl River of Southern Mississippi, but it would do for now. And it offered plenty of room to roam and lots of potential for improvements.

Mother and Daddy would eventually buy hundreds of pine seedlings in Mississippi and plant them in one of the fields. The trees covered several acres. Almost all of them survived and grew tall. The pine tree field held special significance because it was another dream that our parents had of bringing a little bit of Mississippi to bless the terrain. It became a good secluded place to walk, meditate, and relax.

The property came with a large barn. Litters of newborn baby kittens or a brood of baby chickens could sometimes be found in the hay loft of the large barn surrounded by bales or clumps of hay. The barn was also a place to build tunnels or forts out of bales of hay. One could jump into the soft hay lying in the corn crib, or, with enough nerve, jump to the ground from the barn loft.

Rain falling on the red tin roof of the barn, with its compelling pitter-patter, seemed to calm the soul, mesmerizing occupants. An attached shed would serve many purposes over the years but was mostly used to house a tractor and farm implements.

All of the children would learn to safely operate and drive the tractor when they were old enough. We each learned to drive a car in the fields and lanes of the farm. The first turn onto the highway, alone in the car, after receiving your driver's license, was memorable. Driving in the wide fields and down the narrow lane helped us to prepare for real driving.

The barn would shelter, at various times, beef cattle, milk cows, or Mildred's horse, Dude. Mildred loves horses and is a great rider. Dude was a large horse, trained for show, and he could canter. Mildred would saddle and bridle Dude and ride him all over the farm. Ed and I would also learn to ride.

Dude also had a cantankerous streak that he loved to demonstrate. He bit a hole in the upholstery of the front passenger seat of our Plymouth Fury II one day while it was parked with the window open. We were fishing at the time in a boat on the large back pond, one of three ponds. The ponds offered neighborhood kids hours of imaginative play such as seeing who could catch the most minnows or crawdads. Afterward, the captives would always be released unharmed.

The back pond, the field it was in, and the thick woods surrounding it were like a private secluded paradise, and it was a wonderful place for friends and family to gather for picnics, camping, fishing, and games. Few sounds of the outside world or civilization could be heard from here. A few times during the winter months, the pond would freeze solid enough for ice skating.

There were times when three or more cars and the tractor, packed with people and supplies, with the dogs running behind in the dust, would make the trip down the long, long lane to the back pond. The partially shaded lane provided quick and easy access to the very back of the property. It could easily handle most farm equipment and was also an exotic play ground at times.

Mistletoe, blackberry bushes, and persimmon trees that provided a tasty treat when ripe and a bitter sour burst when not ripe lined one side of the lane. The lane, improved and well kept in the past, with a packed dirt surface had been used to train horses pulling sulkies for harness racing.

Thick wooded areas and more than forty acres of pasture clearly separated by several tree lined fences and gates lay in the more than forty acres between the back pond and the house. Several old outbuildings remained on the farm including a smoke house, chicken shed, garage, and outhouse. Bantam chickens and roosters roamed the yard and roosted in the old garage.

The robin's song was sweet music, and the familiar call of the bobwhite quail could often be heard in the pastures as the cocks clearly whistled a bobwhite call to the hens. One might pause for a moment to see if the hens would respond with a bobwhite. Sometimes one of us would call back to them.

A covey of quail or a rabbit could often be flushed from their cover in the fence rows and fields. Songbirds, screech owls, raccoons, possums, and gray squirrels were plentiful as were several kinds of snakes. Foxes, deer, and an occasional bobcat would pass through from time to time. The aroma of honeysuckle filled the air in the long shady lane. The smell of Mr. Gunther's chicken houses, just west of our house, filled the air as well at times, and later, the hogs on the property to the east did the same.

Summertime produced and abundance of blackberries. Picking the blackberries, while trying to avoid the stickers, was always a challenge, but the rewards were great: blackberry cobbler, blackberries with cream, and always blackberry jelly. Mother would work for hours straining those berries and producing the most delicious jelly in the world. We didn't know there was any other kind of jelly. Eventually, we had blueberries too and sometimes dew berries.

Tomato sandwiches were a staple in the summer, together with pineapple sandwiches, fried okra, eggplant, pimento cheese, and fried green tomatoes. There was never enough. We made pizza, cinnamon toast, and doughnuts. There was fresh produce from the garden and canned vegetables and jelly.

When the vegetables in the garden ripened, everyone was called upon for harvest duties. There were peas to shell and corn to shuck. Mother, Gayle, and Mildred would can lots of the vegetables. Deep into autumn, everyone enjoyed watching Ed look for the first snowflake to fall. Snow days were special.

When Ed first began to talk, he called Mildred Neenie, a nickname that has stuck with her. He would call me Bubby. Billy had a few different nicknames for a short amount of time, but none of them really stuck with him. One of the more notable ones came from me when I was very young and apparently very frustrated with him. I called him the worst possible thing my mind could think of at the time. It came out as, "You are a babo demmy crokett dodo."

They tell me that the babo was meant as bad boy. Davy Crockett was a television show of the era but I am not sure why I chose to call him that. The dodo part is self-explanatory. The term stuck for a while mainly because of the humor that came out of the mouth of a small child who actually cherished his big brother.

When we were young, Daddy would ask us, "Can you put your hand on Daddy's man's head?" We each learned to put our hand on our own head. Ed took it a step further one Christmas season when he was about three years old. Daddy was filming Ed while he was standing in front of and facing the Christmas tree. Apparently, there was some significant teasing going on directed toward Ed, and he was pretty disgusted with it and was not putting his hand on his head when prompted. The teasing continued until Ed finally turned around and in a loud voice and demonstrative manner expressed, in no uncertain terms, "I'm Daddy's *man*." Ed was called Man and still is occasionally by Neenie, Bubby, or Billy.

The large front yard was where many activities took place. Long and several acres wide, it was a place of mystery and suspense while playing during the darkness of warm summer evenings. And it was a giant recreation spot at all times.

Friends and family would often gather to relax, talk, and enjoy life in the front yard. Children played frozen tag, hide and seek, croquet, badminton, Hula-Hoops, hopscotch, jump rope, and all sorts of other games. It was also a good place to pitch and catch baseballs, softballs, and footballs and to play wiffle ball.

Large bonfires, especially around Halloween, would light up the night sky. Hot dogs and marshmallows would be attached to a stick or coat hanger and cooked over the fire when the coals were hot. On moonless nights, it was dark and scary. With a full moon, it was still dark but not as scary.

The story of "Speedy" became a Paducah legend and seemed to always be a scary one, but even more so around Halloween. Speedy was a handyman who drowned while fishing in the Ohio River at the Paducah river front. The funeral home director was a friend of Speedy's and decided to experiment with a new powerful preservative he had created. The result was to mummify Speedy's body in almost perfect condition.

He did not give Speedy a pauper's burial but intended to bury him later. Instead, he stood him in a closet for years and occasionally put Speedy on display. He, and his wife, would allow anyone interested to come in and see Speedy in the closet when not on display. This was a test of true courage for the kids of the region.

Speedy's body was washed away during the great flood of 1937 along with much of downtown Paducah. But, miraculously, his body was recovered and returned to the funeral home. It was a very scary tale for the children of the area and many of them remember to this day the time they saw Speedy.

Our Dad did the accounting for the funeral home and would from time to time visit the establishment where he would sit at a table to do his work. He mentioned to us that on a couple of occasions, he was shaken by a loud thud sound in the otherwise quiet and serene funeral home. Upon investigation, he discovered that Speedy had fallen over in the closet.

Speedy later made national and international headlines on television and in print media. He became quite a tourist attraction for a time. Speedy died a pauper but was buried 66 years later as a celebrity. His grave is well marked and still visited in Paducah. Speedy's real name was Charles Atkins.

For those who may not know the exact location of Paducah, I'll take a stab at explaining it the way Billy use to tell his classes. East and west Paducah is about half way between Monkey's Eyebrow and Possum Trot. Yes, they do really exist. No kidding! North and south Paducah is about half way between Memphis and St. Louis. Yes, they also really exist. It's a beautiful small town while also being the largest town in the Jackson Purchase area. It was a great place to grow up in the 1950's through the 1970's.

The Jackson Purchase comprises Kentucky's eight westernmost counties and was once known as the gateway to the west. It is the former tribal home of the Chickasaw Indians and the tract was purchased by the U.S. in 1818 after negotiations by General Andrew Jackson and Governor Isaac Shelby. It is bounded by the Tennessee River to the east, the Ohio River to the north and Mississippi River to the west.

Weekends could often find teenagers driving the approximate one-mile loop around the 19th Hole drive-in, the Dairy Queen drive-in, the bowling alley, and sometimes Noble Park. My first experience of that tradition was with my sister who demanded that I lie down in the backseat so as not to be seen with her as she drove the loop. I could sit up in-between hot spots.

Dialing 808 on the rotary telephone and quickly hanging up would result in a call back ring until someone answered. That was entertainment for a while until parents caught onto the prank and put an emphatic stop to the fun. Though it seemed that every corner had a church, everyone knew that 808 Washington Street was famous for things other than church.

In our front yard, a large bustle about four feet off the ground protruded from one of the majestic oak trees. It was big enough for a child to lie down on and take a nap. There was also a small indentation in the back of the bustle next to the trunk of the tree where one could always find at least one Easter egg. Other assorted objects could sometimes be found there at other times of the year.

Mother and Daddy created one of the best tree swings of all time on a thick limb of one of the giant oaks. The swing was attached with thin nylon ropes to a the long limb, which was at least forty feet off the ground providing plenty of room for giant swings back and forth. It was the source of many fine moments together with friends and family. It was also a place to sit alone and ponder.

During the Christmas season, a tall, thick evergreen tree near the house would beam with the colors of many strands of Christmas lights. At night, the tree stood out as a beacon to the season and could be clearly seen for a good distance by all passersby. The Christmas tree announced the season and proclaimed the beauty and greatness of the birth of the Son of God.

Mildred, like our mother, has a wonderful imagination and could create a world of intrigue and adventure at will. We played outside a lot, day and night, roaming the fields and woods, alone or with friends, when the weather allowed. Colossal sword fights with swords made of tomato stakes sometimes ended badly but the challenge was usually worth the pain.

The stakes also served as more than adequate horses for many adventures. One of our favorite games was playing Ponderosa, imitating the characters on the popular TV program. In another adventure, we pretended we were in Africa on a safari. There were pokeberry and acorn fights and pokeberry ink. A sand pile in the side yard provided hours of entertainment.

There was a magnificent herd of wild horses that roamed the pastures and woodlands. They would come in to view from time to time playfully running and grazing and then disappear for a while. I'm sure they were beautiful. At least that is what Mildred said. She was the only one who could ever seem to see them. Everyone else was either too late to see them or just could not quite see them for some reason.

Occasionally, we could coax Billy into playing some of his western and cartoon movies on his 8 mm home movie projector. He would hang a white sheet in his upstairs bedroom and the projector would cast the image onto the sheet. Sometimes we could talk him into playing the movies backward.

ViewMaster 3D slides were popular for a while, and Mildred would set up slide shows featuring 3D and regular slides of popular cartoons and televisions shows. Billy and Mildred also had a nice and growing collection of 33, 45, and 78 vinyl single records and albums.

We watched the beginning of the British invasion on the family's one black and white television set when the Beatles appeared on the *Ed Sullivan Show*, not fully understanding Mildred's fascination with the group and Paul in particular.

The screened-in front porch was a great place for marbles, jacks, pickup sticks, and the many other games and activities. We threw rocks at bats and hit rocks over the fence with a baseball bat. We can assure you that no bat was ever injured by a rock.

Mildred and I would play cards long after bedtime on the bed under a blanket with a flashlight so as not to disturb anyone. We learned where to step and how to step softly on the upstairs floor late at night to minimize the creaky sound from the wooden floor boards, a sound that must have been magnified to the rooms below. Otherwise, our night would end swiftly and decisively.

A small paddle, with a saying on it, in bright red letters, was prominently displayed in the kitchen. Though we don't remember the words, the context remains vivid. Corporal punishment (spanking) was rarely needed, but when it was, we became familiar with Daddy's belt. If we could talk our way out of the belt, we were directed to go and select a nice, thin switch from one of the large weeping willow trees, which lined the barnyard fence between the house and barn. If you are familiar with the sting of a willow switch, you can understand why we opted for the belt.

The living room was a place to entertain guests and was to be kept in tip-top shape at all times. It also served as Daddy's office at least part of the year until the new office was built, no jumping on the furniture or horseplay or getting the carpet dirty. At least those were the rules. It was a place to celebrate together or to spend time alone pondering the events of life. It was a place to play and a place to rest. There were sad times as we spoke of the death of a relative or friend or discussed other difficult events.

Over the years, the living room would serve the dual purpose of a formal place to meet visitors and then later transform to the central gathering spot for family gatherings. We practiced playing musical instruments and studied schoolwork. We could rehearse Christmas carols and precious hymns as well as the pop tunes of the day.

The living room was at its best when Billy and Gayle lived down the road in Lone Oak and came to visit. They and mother and Mildred and Ed and I would have some of the most memorable times in the living room. We played all sorts of card games, especially bridge. We played board games, Trivial Pursuit, Canasta, Rook, and scrabble while often working a jigsaw puzzle on the side.

Occasionally, after the popcorn ran out, we would head off for midnight red pin bowling to take a break from playing bridge. We went to movies at the drive-in theaters and watched movies like *The Crawling Hand.* We laughed and ate popcorn and sang songs and talked and enjoyed being together. Even when it was not much fun, it was fun just to watch how much fun everyone else was having.

Daddy did not participate much but would hang around and enjoy the activities except when he was trying to sleep. He always seemed to go to bed way too early. He seldom said anything about the level of noise coming from the living room. However, on occasion, we would gather around the piano and sing, which seemed to almost always be after Daddy had gone to bed. There were times when he let us know we needed to pipe down. Mother's favorite song was "My Wild Irish Rose." I do believe she thought of herself as a wild Irish rose.

Christmas day was always celebrated in the living room. There would be a live Christmas tree beautifully decorated with all sorts of precious ornaments and lights. The tree was a cedar or pine tree cut fresh from one of the fields. Mother took pride in decorating the tree and treasured each ornament with which it was adorned. Christmas Eve was always a time of hope and reflection. The number of presents under the tree would slowly increase as Christmas day approached. We rarely got to open a present early, but that seemed to change a little later on.

Eventually, we would fall asleep on Christmas Eve after avoiding the temptation to sneak a peek at the living room. When we awoke, the anticipation built as we waited for Daddy to finish his cup of coffee.

We did not expect to receive a lot for Christmas. But it seemed that Santa always left one or two presents that we had hoped for in addition to the socks and clothes. There was candy in the stockings and chocolate-covered cherries.

When I was about twelve years old, I received a single barrel twenty-gauge shotgun. We each learned to handle and shoot a variety of guns. Safety always came first. We knew to look at what was behind the target and to understand where that shot would end. Every gun should always be considered to be loaded until verified that it was not loaded. Never point the gun at anything that you don't intend to shoot and be considerate of the neighbors.

A race track with race cars was received as a Christmas gift one year. Additional track and cars were added, and a somewhat elaborate race course was constructed in the living room and eventually extending to the dining room and hallway. At one point, the course went under a couch, love seat, and several chairs. The cats would hide under the furniture and race out after the cars as they exited from underneath often chasing the cars around the track and throughout the house.

There were many cats and dogs through the years with names like Colonel, Mabel, Midnight, Sylvester, Pokey, Buttermilk, Lady, Lucky, Buck, Shelia, Heidi, and Butch. Lucky was hit by a car and killed. We learned a little more about the pain of loss as the others would eventually meet their fate. We brought at least one puppy home on the long ride from Mississippi in the car.

On a few occasions, our cattle, the neighbors cattle, or Dude would escape from their fenced confines necessitating a roundup of epic proportions. Neighbors and even strangers driving by would all pitch in to help in the roundup.

One night, a loud scream came from mother's bedroom. "There's someone with a masked face staring at me in the window," she screamed. Everyone quickly rushed to her aide. It seemed that Dude had gotten into the backyard through a hole that had formed in the barnyard fence and was standing outside the house, at the window, looking inside the bedroom.

Mother and Daddy were not pleased at all when the turtle farm Mildred developed in the smokehouse one summer became too successful. It seems at some point that some of the turtles escaped into the garden and were feasting on some of the tomatoes and other fresh vegetables.

It was important to know where everyone was or would be when living on a large farm. In a time before cell phones and GPS, this could be a challenge. One might be in one of the fields, the woods, the lane, or at the back pond. Or they may be in the barn or garden, front yard, at the first pond, in front of the barn, the office, or upstairs.

It was particularly important to establish strict boundaries when playing hide and seek, or the first turn could last until bedtime or suppertime.

In the early sixties, Daddy had the old original pond drained and bulldozers dug a bigger and much deeper pond. He hired a couple of young men to help dig a hole in the bank so the pond would drain into the ditch running through the woods in back of the pond.

Anticipation grew as to what might be at the bottom of that old pond when the water completely drained out. As it turned out, there were more mud puppies at the bottom of the pond than there were fish.

The new pond was ten feet deep with a slope upward in the back. Near completion, while digging in the deep part, the bulldozer struck what turned out to be three springs of water that flowed out of the ground. The bulldozer got stuck, and there was some fear that it might sink out of sight. Another bulldozer came to pull it out, and I believe it got stuck for a while as well.

To this day, that pond is fed by the cold, cold water of those springs. The water level of the pond rarely shrank much even in the hottest of summers. The pond was good for swimming, and one could feel the water becoming ice cold when plunging toward the springs.

The new pond was stocked with largemouth bass, yellow perch, and bluegill. The fishing was excellent for many years, and the bass grew quite large. A ten-foot johnboat was acquired and was used for many years. At that time, we could leave the boat at the pond. But there were strangers who roamed the area hunting, fishing, and doing who knows what else. Mother complained about hunters who did not ask permission before entering the property. At times, we would catch people fishing, and sometimes, they would run off when they saw someone approaching.

This quickly became an outstanding fishing pond and countless hours were spent fishing with family and friends at all times of the day and night. We often left the boat at the pond near the water. One day, we discovered that someone, probably a trespassing hunter, had shot a hole in the bottom of the boat with a rifle. Undaunted, we placed chewing gum in the hole to temporarily stop any leaks and out onto the pond it went. To our amazement, the chewing gum did stop the leak. That was about forty-five years ago, and the gum is still in its place in the boat to this day plugging that hole.

GOD OF GRACE

As I look back on those days, I can now more clearly understand some of the impact that my being born into this family, with the illnesses I would develop, had on my family. I did not understand earlier because it was something I did not want, had not asked for, and did not want to dwell on.

But having a child with serious health problems affects everyone in the family. They demand more attention from the parents. Financial resources intended for the benefit of the entire family are diverted to treat the sick child. This can often exacerbate the harshness of normal sibling rivalries. I did not realize this as a child.

It is a blessing that a child does not often think about the enormous financial burden serious and chronic illness can have on a family or the importance of health insurance and savings accounts to help pay some of the costs of surgeries, physicians, medications, medical equipment, and the many additional expenses of serious chronic illness.

My parents did understand that. And they were able to somehow survive and even prosper at times, even with the enormous medical expenses they incurred as a result of my illnesses. Yet it could have been different if…

To a child, most of these fears seem somehow less cruel. I was fortunate, yes blessed, to have parents and a family that cared for one another and never let me feel sorry for myself.

Don't get me wrong. I learned very early on to run the other way when my mother told me to get in the car but would not tell me where we were going. I lost all those battles and ended up in some of the strangest places.

One was a Catholic hospital in St. Louis where I encountered nuns, sometimes nurses, still dressed in their traditional habit. Five years old and alone, my fear subsided when I discovered that the nun actually knew the Lord's Prayer and said it with me before I fell asleep. They got me into surgery by letting me take the white blanket with me, but I was quite distressed when it did not come out of surgery with me. I did however get a big blue stuffed bear out of that trip.

There was an *Old Yellow* story book in the dresser of the preop room. It became one of my favorite childhood stories. Years later, I learned that the child who owned the book and preceded me into surgery had died at the hospital.

This was not my first brush with death. The first occurred at nine months of age when I was prescribed sulfa drugs to combat asthma and a lingering cold and cough. Sulfa drugs of that time had a different chemical composition than they do now. Apparently, I became dehydrated, and the sulfa crystallized in my kidneys causing permanent damage to both kidneys. The doctors realized that the damage would cause kidney failure and, most likely, death at some point. This was a time before dialysis and transplantation, making the long-term outlook bleak at best.

The second life-altering event occurred while my mother was working on folding clothes, and I saw what

I thought were grapes in a dish on the dresser. I picked up a handful and put them in my mouth. Don't laugh, I loved grapes and probably jumped at the opportunity. They were actually small pearl beads from a broken necklace. She noticed immediately that I had put them in my mouth and quickly made me spit them out. But I had swallowed one bead, and it was stuck in my windpipe.

I am told that it then quickly became a life-and-death struggle. I was rushed to the local doctor who tried to grasp the lone remaining bead with an instrument and pull it from my windpipe. The instrument was too large, and the bead was pushed further down where it aspirated into my lung, making the situation much more desperate. In a time before interstate highways, my parents made the long and arduous 140-mile journey to Vanderbilt University Hospital where I was then rushed into surgery. Our family friend, Georgia Mae, came to Paducah from Mississippi to care for Billy and Mildred during that time.

The lower lobe of my right lung was removed, and the rest of the lung had received damage from the prior attempts to remove the bead and by the bead itself. After the surgery, I contracted pneumonia, and with all the other complications, recovery was not certain. I was in the hospital for several weeks. The result was a lifelong battle with lung disease.

The relationship with Vanderbilt is a long one. In 1983, I underwent surgery to repair several abdominal hernias that had developed in the surgical incision area since transplant. The procedure was repeated on a more extensive basis by the transplant team at Georgetown University Hospital in 2004.

My right lung collapsed on three separate occasions in 1987 and 1988 with a spontaneous pneumothorax. The third time, I was transported back to Vanderbilt where the transplant team consulted with the pulmonary team to determine what further treatment may be available.

At one point, I was evaluated by Dr. Bill Frist, a renowned heart-lung transplant surgeon. Dr. Frist would later become a two-term United States senator representing Tennessee. Chemical pleurodesis with instillation of tetracycline was subsequently performed in my right lung in an effort to avoid recurrence of the lung collapsing.

I have often recalled the story my mom told about praying in the Vanderbilt Hospital Chapel when I was in surgery after swallowing the bead. After much prayer, she began to sing a hymn: "God of Grace and God of Glory…grant us wisdom grant us courage for the facing of this hour, for the facing of this hour." The words of that song have been my own prayer on several distressing occasions throughout life.

I am told that the surgery and subsequent events were described by one of the doctors in an article published in a medical journal. Ed and I were the subject of another medical journal article after the transplant.

Not much was known about lung disease or asthma in that day and time. There were some medications such as Tedral. But everything considered, the doctor said I probably would not live to be eleven. I did not know that he had told my parents that until years later. I just wanted to be normal with a normal country boy's childhood.

Another secret trip removed my tonsils and yet another yielded some type of surgery that remains a mystery to me to this day. There were many visits to the West McCracken County Clinic for breathing related issues. Dr. Charles Harting, a graduate of the Heath High School class of 1933, founded the Clinic in 1953 and operated it in this rural community until 1972.

The embarrassment, particularly to a child with a chronic illness, may be devastating. I had quite a bit of experience with this aspect. As a child, on a Cub Scout trip to St. Louis, I suddenly became the center of unwanted attention when I became dizzy and sick with asthma. It seems my condition put a damper on the trip equaled only by the long, dark rainy trip home.

Our high school band traveled one year to Washington, DC, to participate in the Cherry Blossom Festival Parade. Though only an eighth grader, I was selected to travel with the band. The usual anxiety was heightened by the fear that somehow I would mess this up too with some type of weird sickness. All went well that time.

I totally fainted at a grave side funeral in the heat of a Mississippi summer afternoon. My uncle was burying his wife, daughter, and grandson who had been killed in a head-on car crash. Yes, unwanted attention yet again.

This uncle was a unique man of faith. As a Gideon, he placed Bibles in hotel rooms and other places where someone who needed an infusion of faith and courage may find it. He suffered so many tragedies that I could barely know what to say to him. He seemed strong but worn-down.

Another one of his daughters was savagely raped and murdered in her apartment in Biloxi, Mississippi. Though law enforcement knew who had done it, Hurricane Camille had destroyed all the evidence. A young son died in a freak bicycle accident, and yet another son had died young of a rare cancer disease. Despite all of the tragedy, he endured. He was a pleasant man to be around and was a keeper of the faith and of our family history.

I had several trips to the barbershop cut short by dizziness. One day, at fourteen years of age, I decided to ride my bike over to the barbershop to get a haircut. While in the barber chair, I became faint and nearly passed out. The barber, a family friend, took me and my bicycle home. My parents were exasperated with what seemed to be no solutions to the never-ending health problems. They had tried everything they knew about to restore my health.

This started a chain of events that led to a lengthy hospitalization. I still have flashbacks and much unease each and every time I get my hair cut.

They decided to take me to Dr. Baird whose home and office was in the tiny rural town of Bandana, Kentucky. Dr. Baird was somewhat of an old country doctor and had graduated from the University of Mississippi. He was trusted by his patients and loved in the small community.

After examination, he recommended that I be taken to Baptist Memorial Hospital in Memphis, Tennessee, as soon as possible. I spent the days in bed at home while waiting to travel to the hospital in Memphis. I remember the somber mood around the house because I was so weak and the future so uncertain. Mildred came into the room, after talking to my parents. We made eye contact, but neither spoke. She could only kneel down by the bed and cry. For the first time in a long time, I became very scared.

During the three weeks I spent at Baptist and LeBohner's Children's Hospital in Memphis, the doctors confirmed that the immediate concern was controlling chronic pulmonary disease. But they confirmed that my kidneys were failing and that I would probably not live to twenty-four years of age. Dialysis and kidney transplant was in its infancy, rare, and expensive. I was fourteen at the time and had thus exceeded predictions that I would not live to age eleven.

Many years later, my wife and I rushed our youngest daughter to LeBohner's Children's Hospital, after she had apparently swallowed some of my mom's medication. Karen, the girls, and I were living in Memphis, and my mom was visiting with us for a few days and helping with the babysitting and house chores while Karen and I were at work. It was a scary situation for all of us, and it was very difficult to watch as the doctors pumped Jennifer's stomach. She recovered quickly and apparently had not taken much, if any, of the medication.

Once again, I was blessed. Life returned to that of a normal teenager. School, sports, friends, and family were only interrupted by allergy shots, percussion and nebulizer treatments, oxygen therapy, and endless medications.

I had learned to pace myself. I could play much longer if I exerted myself more evenly over a long period instead of using all my energy up quickly. This was important because our family was a sports-loving family. I had to keep up with my sister and brothers who were always involved in something.

But there was no pain. And I could do almost anything, often against the advice or knowledge of my parents, if I paced myself properly. And almost no one knew that I had been sick or had a chronic condition. I tried not to think of it much. Gayle would often drive me to Dr. Baird's for twice weekly allergy shots until I was old enough to drive.

My parents did have to renovate the upstairs of our home in an attempt to create a dust-free room because of the pulmonary issues. They made three rooms from what had been an open area. My small room was intended to be sterile with nothing in it but a bed. I did add a small television and my sister's record player.

Challenged as a youngster, I quickly learned to live life as full and long as possible. How could I complain about my circumstances when so many people endure much worse? I often recalled what my mother would sometimes say to me when I would ask, "Why me?" She would tell me of someone suffering much more and say, "There but for the grace of God go I."

My wife, Karen, and I were walking through Johns Hopkins Hospital one day after a doctor visit. As we passed the gift shop, we paused and then purchased a stuffed bear not unlike the one I received when in the hospital at age five. We took the elevator to the children's floor and asked the nurses if they knew of a child who might be uplifted by this gift. They thought and quickly said yes.

We went to the room of an eight-year-old boy who was lying in bed. His mom was sitting in a chair by his bedside. His shaven head made his eyes seem bigger and brighter, and his smile radiated as he realized, after a quizzical stare, that the bear was for him. We were told that he did not have many more weeks to suffer in this world, but that the bear had brightened his day. That is not the first or last time we had done that. Each time we give in that manner, we remember the cards and letters and words of encouragement that had been so encouraging to us.

TAX TIME AND FLOWER GARDENS

A large double-sided sign at one end of the long circular gravel driveway in front of the house advertised my dad's accounting business and announced a new season of tax time.

When the family moved to Kentucky and bought this ponderosa, Daddy worked as a pipe fitter at the power plant being built to supply power to the gaseous diffusion plant that was also being built nearby. To earn extra money, he set up a desk in the small living room of our home and prepared the tax returns of some of the people who worked at the plant. His business education and the accounting experience received from his job in Washington, DC, was about to propel him into a very successful new career.

To supplement this income, Daddy traveled around the region for two or three summers to sell crop insurance to the many farmers of the region. And because he too was a small farmer and a businessman, he could easily relate to the unique tax situations of the farmers and small business owners in the region. He quickly earned their trust, and the business that had begun in our home grew quite quickly. He was soon able to leave his job at the plant and grow his own business full time.

The business soon outgrew the living room, and additions were made to the house. A utility room, garage, and nice size office was built. During tax time between January and April, the driveway would often be filled with cars as people arrived to discuss their tax business and return later to pick up their completed federal, state, and, in some cases, business tax returns.

We had a telephone party line for a while. After the office was built, we had two lines, one for the house and one for the office. They had distinctive rings so you could tell a business call from personal. One could also tell the difference between the office doorbell and the house doorbell.

A buzzer was installed in the office behind mother's desk. It would ring in the house. I believe one ring was for Billy, though he was away from home by the time the buzzer was installed, two for Mildred, three for Tom, and four for Ed. One should respond quickly when buzzed. Multiple buzzes usually meant "Quit fighting and keep the noise down or your father is going to come into the house and you don't want that to happen!"

Daddy worked late into the night during tax time. Mother was an essential part of the tax business working only during tax time. She greeted customers, answered the phone, worked numerous tax returns, distributed them to customers picking up their returns, filed, answered all sorts of questions, and much more. They had many friends as clients and would engage in all kinds of conversation.

Mother would often go on strike in January at the beginning of tax time holding out for higher pay from Daddy than she had received the year before. Sometimes she would hold out as long as February before the issue was resolved. I think they enjoyed the contest much more than their children did, but we were told not to worry, and sure enough, either she or Daddy always gave in and reached a compromise solution.

The business continued to grow, and several employees were added during tax season. They did not become wealthy by any means, but our parents sent all of their children to college. They attended and supported their church and were active in the community. I am forever thankful for the sacrifice my parents made. When I see the wonderful people their grandchildren and great-grandchildren have become, I know their sacrifice was worth it. I am also thankful for my country and her veterans who secured for them the opportunity to pursue and achieve a better life for themselves and their children.

All of Daddy's children grew up around the office, and his clients, helping out when we could, especially during the busiest days of tax season. Billy worked for him for a couple of years at night while teaching high school during the day. All of the children learned to prepare tax returns, at least, at a minimum, the more simple ones. We learned a lot about customer service and treating people with courtesy and respect while observing Mother and Daddy in the office. Our parents treated people with patience and goodness well after the rest of the world ceased to treat the same people with patience and goodness.

Ed remembered that, "Daddy would leave the house, sometimes at odd hours, to visit and take care of a friend who was an alcoholic. I think sometimes he did this to be with him so that he wouldn't drink and sometimes to tend to him after he had been drinking. It seems that when I asked Mother why he did this, she told me that everyone else had given up on Charlie but not Daddy and that doing things like that was part of what made him a good man."

Mildred told, "A kind and gentle man who seldom raised his voice or uttered criticisms or displeasure. When he did, we knew he had strong feelings about whatever it was that produced the passion. He would sit at the table drinking coffee and reading. From time to time, he would chuckle about something. I loved hearing him chuckle. It is still one of my favorite things of all. He seemed to me to be a man of few words, but I loved it when he gave me advice about something or told me about his life and the things that meant something to him, the things he had experienced. I truly wish I had just talked to him more than I did."

Ed told the story of coming home from a date one fall Saturday night to find our yard had been TP'D. "I was usually, with my friends, the perpetrator of such events and not the victim. After all, who in his right mind would attempt to TP a house where at least one Doberman resided? And at the time we had two Dobermans! However, they were both in the dog pen when I got home.

"When I asked Daddy how this happened, he told me that Richard Montgomery called and asked him if he would put the dogs up for a little while, which Daddy agreed to do. I told him the only reason Richard would ask him to do that was so that he could TP our yard, to which Daddy responded, 'I know that. I figured he owed you at least one.'"

Daddy retired a few months before the transplant took place. If he had not been retired, the transplant would not have been scheduled in February since that would be one of the busiest months of the tax season.

Daddy was the first president of the Kentucky Association of Accountants. He was an enrolled agent licensed to practice and represent clients before the Internal Revenue Service and he held a U.S. Treasury card. He was a Kentucky Colonel, served several years as manager of Khoury League baseball teams, and was an active member of the Concord Lions Club and the Grahamville Masonic Lodge. Mother and Daddy were charter members and organizers of Concord United Methodist Church. He was a member of the Disabled American Veterans.

Upon his death, the Kentucky Association of Accountants published the following resolution.

Be It Resolved: That in the death of William B. Cooper, the Kentucky Association of Accountants and the Accounting Profession in general have lost a dear friend, a landmark, and an ardent professional accountant. Bill was the first enrolled accountant in the "Purchase" area and the first active President of K.A.A. We mourn with his loved ones at the passing of Bill and rejoice with them in the certain knowledge that we shall be with him again when we present our earthly records for audit. Be it further resolved that this resolution be placed in the minutes of K.A.A and published in the bulletin and that a copy be sent to Mrs. Cooper with our sincere condolences and respect.

I suppose Mother and Daddy always had a vegetable garden, if at all possible. Corn, tomatoes, okra, beans, peas, green peppers, potatoes, peanuts, and other staples would be planted and harvested. It is a lot of work to successfully maintain a garden, especially one that large, but the payoff was well worth the effort. Mother was a great cook, and when she prepared fresh produce from the garden, it was a meal fit for kings. Jars of canned vegetables from the garden, jellies, and fruit were stored in the basement for enjoyment later in the year.

Each spring, the garden would need to be prepared by plowing and disking the ground when it was dry enough from the winter freeze. However, in our family, tax time ruled over everything else, and it lasted from January until the April 15 deadline and beyond. Tax time was when a significant amount of the family income was earned. Since Mother worked in the family business too during tax time, she rarely had time to work in the garden at all until after tax time.

Flowers, shrubs, and bushes of all kinds displayed an incredible and beautiful mixture of colors in numerous flower beds, around the house, and yard. Mother had a special gift for flower gardening. She planted and cared for her creations tirelessly, and the results of her creative beauty were enjoyed and admired by many who drove by our beautiful yard.

She put a lot of thought into what went where as she planted each bulb and seedling, and the result was spectacular. She planted dogwoods, red buds, azaleas, and almost everything that could grow. These were highlighted by the weeping willow trees and several pine trees. One of her greatest sources of pride was her rose garden. She had the traditional colors of roses as well as some new varieties of color, which made it a sight to behold.

Mother was the definition of a country girl. But she was also a lady who could mix and hobnob with the crusty when necessary. But she and Daddy were both most comfortable in the country. They did not put on airs or suffer fools easily.

THROUGH THICK AND THIN

ONE FAMILY STORY

> Families are the backbone of our country. They are the stability, the comfort, the safety, the haven where parents should raise their children in love and peace. Home should be a place where one feels accepted, nurtured, cared for, and above all, it should be a place of safety. Home should be a refuge from pressures of life – work, social obligations, school, and peer pressure.
>
> Families should strengthen churches, and churches should strengthen our nation. Something has gone terribly wrong. Families are broken, churches are broken, and our nation has forsaken the principles upon which it was founded: principles of honor, respect, truth, loyalty, decency, courage, a deep appreciation of freedom and of its price.
>
> —Mildred Cooper Russell

I suppose that it really is true that, for most of us, if we survive to adulthood, even without any serious illness, that it could only be by the grace of God. There are so many obstacles to overcome and near-miss accidents as we make our way through life.

That was certainly the case for me whether it was occasionally racing way to fast on a deserted highway or jumping off of roofs or even challenging a massive nest of wasps just to prove courage.

Ed had his share of incidents as well. I was there for some of them. We were almost always together doing something. I was very happy to have a baby brother when he was born, and seven years younger than I seemed the perfect separation of age. Mildred, on the other hand, was hoping for a baby sister but recovered from the disappointment and has always loved him very much.

The four of us had many wonderful and memorable times together. I had the best of both worlds. Since I was in the middle, age-wise, I experienced years of wonderful times together with each of them. And Billy and Gayle were right there in the mix for a lot of it.

One time, I was mowing grass with the push mower out beside the old garage. Ed, who was about eight at the time, was playing near the old smokehouse a few yards away but within eye sight. From the corner of my eye, I saw him awkwardly fall to the ground and noticed that he had a very odd look on his face. I walked over and noticed a considerable amount of blood coming out of his leg in the thigh.

I picked him up and carried him into the house and told Daddy, who was on the couch napping and watching television, that Ed had been hurt. He and Mom immediately went into action and rushed Ed to the emergency room. I noticed blood on the sleeve of my shirt in the front elbow area and knew that the projectile had penetrated all the way through his leg. I called Billy and Gayle who were still living in Lone Oak at the time.

The doctor treating Ed at the emergency room said it was a gunshot wound. There were often hunters in the woods around our house, and this was apparently a stray rifle bullet that had hit Ed. He was on crutches for several weeks but, except for two scars, fully recovered.

Another time, on a cold winter day, we were upstairs, and Ed was about to climb out the window onto the long, slanted roof to retrieve something. There was a coating of ice on the roof mixed with some snow. I told Ed that it was not a good idea to climb out on the roof. He might slide, gathering steam as he went, and slide right off the roof onto the ground. He tried it anyway, and as he was completely out the window, he began to slide. I quickly grasped the hood of the jacked he was wearing and pulled him back in.

And there were other times, like when I accidentally hit him in the head with a baseball bat or when he fell, hands first, into the ashes of a Halloween pit fire in the front yard and another emergency room visit after a bicycle accident. The bicycle accident occurred while Ed was attempting to dribble a basketball down the road to a friend's house while pedaling. He actually accomplished the feat until the tires hit some loose gravel.

Much of our time was spent playing baseball, football, and endless hours of wiffle ball. We did a lot of exploring on our little slice of heaven. When the chest-high grass in the large field we were traveling in was too tall for him, I carried him on my shoulders, usually with

Buck, our German shepherd, clearing the path ahead of all potential enemies.

I was walking a path through one of the pastures one day with Buck smelling the path a few feet in front of me. At one point, he turned and positioned himself directly in front of me so that I could not go forward. At first, I thought he was being playful, so I tried to step around him. He moved to position himself in front of me again. I got the message this time and cautiously surveyed the ground ahead of us. Sure enough, there was a big old snake just lying there waiting for me to step on him. I thanked Buck profusely, and we took a different path.

We would all go to the basement of the house during tornado warnings. Over the years, some of the dogs would hesitate to go with us, but we could usually manage to get them down there. The cats were another story. If you could find them, you dare not pick them up and try to carry them down the stairs into the basement or a fate worse than the tornado warning was certain!

During the Cuban Missile crisis of October 1962, Mother built a fallout shelter in the basement. The country took the event very seriously. She used wood, brick, cinder block, sheet metal, and other things to construct a small crude shelter for the family. The crisis was the closest the Soviet Union and United States came to nuclear war and assured mutual destruction. Ed was only two and maybe too young to remember, but it certainly got the attention of Mildred and me.

A loud scream came from Mother's room one afternoon. We all rushed in, and she was standing next to her chest of drawers with a stunned look of horror. She had reached into the top drawer to retrieve her reading glasses when the arm of the glasses started moving. She realized it was a snake and screamed.

Ed had a coonskin cap that somehow ended up in Daddy's chair in the utility room where he napped and watched TV. Daddy was about halfway seated when he noticed what he thought was a cat that he was about to sit on. He made his best effort but could not stop and voiced his displeasure loudly as he was sure he had just smashed the cat. The fact that it was a coonskin cap and not a cat did not ease his immense displeasure for quite some time.

Climbing as close as possible to the top of a tall tree was a skill that we would each learn through trial and error. The thrill of hiding in a tree or enjoying a panoramic view of the territory can be an irresistible challenge to youngsters. One quickly learns, however, that climbing up a tree is much easier than climbing back down. I can sympathize with the stories of a cat that is stuck in a tree.

Though we were never stuck, one of Mildred's friends did get stuck in the tree house built in a sycamore tree by the first pond. She was able to climb up the tree to the tree house, but she could not climb back down. Upon realizing this, she became frightened and began screaming at the top of her lungs. Mildred and I were afraid that her parents, and ours, would hear her frantic screams and think something awful had happened. No amount of coaxing or coaching could quiet her or convince her to even try to make the journey down. After a few moments, Billy appeared, much to our relief. He, in his gentle voice and manner, was able to guide our friend down from the tree. We were worn out from the emotion of it but relieved that the problem had been resolved without parental involvement.

Summer night noises could be both enchanting and frightening. They were mostly comforting and pleasant, but there were times when they added an element of unease to a situation we found ourselves in. Friday nights would find Mildred and me watching Shock Theater and other scary shows on late-night television. For a time, the television was on our enclosed front porch.

After the show was over and the TV was quiet, it was time for us to go upstairs to bed. We usually did not make the move right away because we were still processing the scary scenes, imagining all kinds of personal danger. It was the perfect setting for night noises to contribute to our heightened awareness of our surroundings. We often made the journey upstairs slowly, conquering one room at a time.

The sump pump in the basement sometimes sounded like something from Shock Theater and caused more than a few chilling moments. On more than one occasion, the slow journey upstairs was halted by the sudden action of the sump pump. The sump pump drained water that had accumulated on the floor of the basement. If you have never heard one, I don't know how you can understand the sound it made. It sounded like a person groaning, sort of in slow motion, and distorted.

This sound, after just watching a particular scary show, could practically stop our hearts. Everyone else in the house was asleep, so we had to endure and survive these events without making much noise. In spite of this, we continued to watch Shock Theater every week.

In addition, there were plenty of unexplainable phenomena in that old house and the surrounding fields. Not all of it was childhood imagination. But we did have our ways of explaining the unexplainable, much to our parents' chagrin. Crazy Chambers was mostly in the woods surrounding the back pond though he could appear anywhere. He was to be feared and avoided at all costs. He was a real person, and we believed he had murdered his wife. There were several anxious occasions where it was deemed wiser to leave the location than to risk the ire of Crazy Chambers. All of us at one time or another had an experience that included Crazy Chambers. I cannot remember for sure, but I think he was simply a slightly mentally challenged person who liked to roam around in the woods.

Mae inhabited the upstairs wraparound closet for a short time. Though her exact appearance remains a mystery, her mannerisms could probably best be explained as somewhat akin to that of a wicked witch, and her characteristics and sudden appearance on the scene is the easiest to explain of all the phantoms. Mae was the name of the wife of a radio disc jockey upon whom Mildred and her friend Linda had a serious crush. Mae was the instigator of several unfortunate incidents revolving around Mildred, Ed, and me.

A much more sinister figure was known to us by the name Mad Myrtle. She could materialize in a number of places. Havoc and mayhem of some kind almost always accompanied her. It was prudent to try and understand her intentions and appease her when possible. It was often necessary to first determine, after much discussion, if the situation was the result of Mad Myrtle or Mae.

Mad Myrtle was revealed around a Girl Scout camp fire by one of the troop leaders. Mildred used all kinds of things like this to her advantage, especially to manipulate and frighten her younger brothers, but she was often the victim of her own overactive imagination.

The most terrifying of all the apparitions, by far, was Hawkins. He was not restricted to the upstairs wraparound closet as was Mae. And though Mad Myrtle could be quite terrifying, her intentions seemed to be more of those of a pest than an evil combatant. There were a couple of times when we questioned if she had actually saved us from some of the more serious consequences of a sinister plot that Hawkins was perpetrating upon us.

Hawkins was not to be taken flippantly. I suppose he could best be described as a type of shape-shifting prankster, a sort of vampire, with a very dark side and a mysterious but distinct aura. Mildred was the one most adept at detecting his presence and intent. She trained me to do the same, and we did our best to educate a somewhat disbelieving and annoyed Ed, who did in fact master the ability. Billy, Mother, and Daddy however seemed to be too suspicious of motive to fully acquire the gift of recognition or appreciate the significance of the subject.

I am not actually sure how the name Hawkins was derived. It could have been from one of the characters in the countless scary movies we watched. He became a big part of our activities around the neighborhood and was especially useful in controlling younger, more easily frightened folk.

Hawkins was viewed in human form mostly at the back pond, in the thick woods and pasture surrounding the pond, in the barn, and in the wraparound closet upstairs. He was, however, most commonly invisible even to the trained and vigilant eye. Though not a demon, he could inhabit the bodies of animals for a short time, but there is no evidence that he has the capability to possess the human body even briefly.

One of Hawkins's most troublesome characteristics was his unique ability to travel rapidly and show up almost anywhere usually at the most inconvenient of times. Even today, there are instances when an event transpires that will cause Mildred, Ed, and me to pause and, if we happen to be together at the time, exchange a knowing glance that this occurrence has to be the work of Hawkins.

Blaming Hawkins for little incidents and quirky things that happened was a daily thing at our house. We were very hard on Ed, using the threat of Hawkins doing harm to him to try to get him to do what we did or did not want him to do. After a few years of this, our parents became tired of it and told us to quit talking about Hawkins. This was due in large part to Ed's complaining and noncooperation. Finally in exasperation, Mother told us never to mention his name again.

Mildred, who could not resist taking things to the limit and beyond, would soon break the rule. One summer evening, Mildred, Ed, and I were playing cards at the table. Mother had left strict instructions before going to bed that there should be no noise and don't pick on or upset Ed with talk about Mad Myrtle or ghosts. But in the normal course of affairs, the loving bantering went back and forth.

Ed was winning, continually. This was not acceptable. At one point, he was promised that if he did not settle down and play right that, exactly at midnight, Hawkins was going to attack his cat that was sleeping on the nearby couch. This would be a sign that he should be afraid of Hawkins and his power. Ed was incredulous. He reminded us of what Mother had said. We continued to push him. He threatened to tell Mother.

At exactly midnight, to everyone's astonishment, the cat jumped up and began choking and coughing feverishly, seemed like he was going to die, and suddenly ran away. Everyone became amazed, stunned, and very concerned, and the look on Ed's face was priceless. Mildred then, being in her element, said, "See, we told you Hawkins would get your cat."

He began hollering, "Mom, Mom, Hawkins is killing my cat!" He ran to her bedroom, and a sense of doom began to settle upon us.

When Mother came into the den, she gave us a severe tongue-lashing. Mildred, still not having learned her lesson, blurted out, "We didn't do anything, honestly, it was Hawkins." At this point, I thought we were destined to sleep in the barn. I believe Mother mentioned that in no uncertain terms. The thought of that, after what we had just witnessed, was a punishment of its own. It was a mercy that the attention was given back to the cat. He was found and had recovered.

Mildred and I restrained ourselves for quite a while after that episode. We feared being given Castor Oil, one of Mother's favorite remedies. She believed that bad behavior was due to constipation, thus Castor Oil. We will never understand how she could embrace such a baseless theory. If the offense occurred during the day, we might have to cut a willow switch for ourselves. Nothing compares to the sting of a willow switch!

Late one night, as we all slept, loud, terrifying screams came from an upstairs bedroom where Mildred and one of her friends were spending the night. Mother and Daddy rushed to see what crisis could be causing such panicked screams. They had seen a clown staring at them from a window on the roof!

Their bed was under a window in the front part of the upstairs. The clown was on the roof in the back of the house looking in a window directly across from them. This caused quite a scramble, and the yard and surroundings were extensively searched. No stranger was found. Everyone was skeptical as to whether they had actually seen a clown. This could be just another joke that the two were known for. But they both insisted, and do to this day, that they did each see the clown.

None of us can understand how we survived the Christmas Ed got a minibike. It just happened that a heavy snow blanked the ground on Christmas Eve and on Christmas day that year. But that could not dampen the family's enthusiasm. We all took turns navigating the minibike through the snow. At one point, we hooked the sled to the back of the minibike with what was about a ten-foot rope, and off we went.

I was driving, and Ed was on the sled as we maxed out the speed, headed past the barn through the barnyard, and down the narrow lane. The sled was twisting and turning in what was a fabulous ride. But it is hard to stop a minibike on a dime in the snow on a narrow lane with your brother tethered behind on a sled. Just a few scrapes and bruises and a wonderful time had by all.

BASEBALL

Billy and Mildred had been very active in the Methodist Youth Fellowship (MYF), Boy Scouts, and Girl Scouts. And they loved baseball. Baseball was always important to our entire family. I played the second year of atom league baseball and two years of bantam league. The atom league manager did not return, and Daddy took over as manager. I played third base and first base. I was on the high school baseball team my junior year.

Ed played atom, bantam, and midget league with Daddy as the manager. Ed could play any position but excelled as a pitcher and usually played second when not pitching. I was a coach for the team. Bill's Pharmacy was the sponsor of the team and the team's name. Ed also played league ball after that and was a pitcher on the high school team. Mildred was an outstanding softball player. She played in many of the pickup games we played in the field in front of the barn.

There was a moment in Ed's very first game that is still a very vivid memory for both of us. One of the umpires did not show up. I was asked if I would umpire in the field when our team was at bat. Although I was also the first base coach, I reluctantly agreed to fill in as umpire as well. In the third inning, Ed smashed a clean single to right field, his very first hit in organized baseball. He had a nice smile on his face and, as coach, I complimented him as he reached first and rounded the bag.

Then I noticed, as coach, that the ball was thrown to the first baseman. He did not return the ball to the pitcher but retained the ball surreptitiously in his glove for an attempt at the old hidden ball trick. Ed was two or three steps off of first and, as coach, I emphatically but with a low voice said a couple of times "get back, get back on base." Then the first baseman tagged Ed and, as umpire, I somewhat reluctantly but convincingly called him out. Our eyes met and the astonished and gloomy look on his face matched the dejection on my face. I think everyone else in attendance had a nice little laugh at the state of affairs as they realized the irony of the situation. His first hit became one that the two of us would always remember.

Mother kept the official score card for our team at each game. These games brought the family together during the summer for practices and games in a way no other activity could. Some things about the games and Daddy stick out in Ed's memory.

"Are you sure about that, Mr. Umpire?" often Daddy was addressing a fifteen- or sixteen-year-old kid but still referred to him as Mr. Umpire.

"Any pitch below the knees and above the armpits is a bad pitch."

"Run, son! Run! Don't watch the ball!" (While that was often directed at me, it could have been anyone on the team. At the ballpark, we were all his sons.)

From a crouch at the edge of the dugout, I would hear him tell me to "Pull the string." It was more than a signal to throw my changeup. It was a statement. "We've got him right where we want him. Now finish him off."

I suppose Daddy had loved baseball from an early age. He became a Washington Senators fan while living in Washington, DC, and attended several games. He was privileged to see Babe Ruth and other great legends of the game play baseball.

The Saint Louis Cardinals baseball radio network could be heard throughout the south and midwest all the way to the Rocky Mountains. In those days, Dizzy Dean lived in Bond, Mississippi, only a few miles from Purvis. I can remember Daddy driving by the house to show me where he lived. Dizzy and his brother Paul played for the Cardinals on a championship team known as the Gashouse Gang.

I picked up on Billy's love for the game, the Cardinals, and Stan Musial. I remember listening to the last three games of the 1963 season as the Cardinals almost won the pennant. That was also Stan the Man's last season. They won the World Championship in 1964 beating the Yankees in seven games. Daddy, Billy, Ed, and I drove to Saint Louis in 1967 to see the Cardinals play Saturday and Sunday games. We stayed overnight in Saint Louis, also a treat.

A client friend of Daddy's would organize bus trips to see the Cardinals play a few times each summer. Mother, Daddy, Ed, and I went on several of those day trips. Ed and I went on other trips with Laurie's dad Jim and Don Hayes, a dear friend of Ed and our family. Ed and his family have made several trips over the years to see the Cardinals play.

Our front yard on the left side of the house extended from in front of the barn to the road. This provided an area large enough to play softball or baseball or football and all sorts of other sports related activities. A strong male would have to hit a baseball solidly to hit it over the road on a fly, and it was done a few times. A square section of one-inch board about the size of a strike zone was nailed to the barn and used as a target for pitching when no catcher was available.

At times, we could organize as many as twelve or more kids from the neighborhood into teams for a game. Over the years, several of those friends have mentioned what great memories they have of those days playing in that field. It was shaped more for football than baseball, but we always seemed to make it work.

Adjacent to the baseball field was a basketball goal with a grass court. Billy had put a post in the ground and nailed a wooden backboard to the post. The backboard would eventually need to be replaced, and another post was added to help stabilize the backboard. It was not easy to get an honest bounce from the ball, yet we managed to have some good competition at times with several children and adults participating in games. Many hours were spent alone shooting hoops and dreaming of making the last shot of a Heath Pirate or a University of Kentucky basketball victory.

Daddy could often be seen hitting fly balls to Ed or me in the field in front of our barn, a task he seemed to greatly enjoy. Ed and I would practice pitching, hitting, and fielding for hours in the front yard, in the field in front of the barn, or anywhere we happened to be. Bill's Pharmacy pitchers, and sometimes position players, would come to our house for extra practice on the ball field a few times each summer.

Daddy was selected to be manger of the region's all-star baseball team one summer. Ed and a couple of other

Bill's Pharmacy teammates were selected for the team, and I was one of the coaches. The competition was an elite all-star team from Southern Illinois. Our team consisted of the top players from teams that we had competed with for years, which made the event much more enjoyable. The score of the game was close to the very end but ended with a victory for the other team.

We would frequently pick up and take home team members who needed a ride to practice or games. Herb Chapman was the shortstop on the Bill's Pharmacy team. We would pick up Herb on our way to practice or games many times, and quite often his younger brother Stevie would come with him. Stevie would sometimes serve as the batboy for the team.

Herb's mother would often sit with our mom at the games. She would fill in as official score keeper when Mom was not there. Their father, an excellent musician in his own right, owned a music shop at their home.

It was easy to see from an early age the musical talent of the two brothers. They both went on to have exceptional careers as musicians, singers, and songwriters. Steven Curtis Chapman would become one of the greatest Christian recording artists of all time.

Baseball, softball, volleyball, and other sports continue to be an important part for each of our families. Ed and Laurie played in an elite fast-pitch softball league for years, and Ed played on several basketball teams. Each of their children played high school sports, and Clay received numerous scholarship offers to play college baseball. Our daughter Kelly played recreational soccer, basketball, and one year of high school softball. Younger daughter Jenny played several years of youth league basketball.

Karen, our two little girls, and I lived in Colorado in 1993 when the Colorado Rockies Major League baseball team played the first game of their inaugural season. I was able to acquire thirty-four tickets for the first ever Rockies baseball game played at Mile High Stadium. More than eighty-three thousand people attended the game, which is the largest crowd to ever see a baseball game. All but our four tickets were for coworkers at the training center where I worked and their families. Our four tickets were two rows from the field near first base in temporary bleacher seats used to accommodate the huge crowd for that one game only.

In the fourth inning, Alex Cole of the Rockies hit a grounder to third and the Montreal third baseman's throw to first sailed over the first baseman's head and out of play under the temporary seats where we were sitting. Karen retrieved the game ball, which was later autographed by the Rockies manager and the principal owner. It was a great pleasure to take the family to several Rockies games each season, but the scene was quite bewildering at times when they played the Cardinals. We also attended the first ever game of the Colorado Avalanche Hockey team and the Colorado Rapids soccer team.

We become fans of the Washington Nationals while living in Virginia, attending several games, including the first ever played at Nationals Park. Though we have enjoyed cheering for the Rockies and Nationals as loyal fans, our allegiance to the Cardinals has never wavered.

DEVASTATION AND DESPAIR

An army of bulldozers and huge earthmovers approached our property line one day in the summer of 1969. Mother and Ed were there waiting. Mother stood with a shotgun directly in the path of the bulldozer preventing it from breaching the boundary line onto our private property. She refused all requests to move, and the county sheriff was called to the scene. He was kind and understanding and finally said, "June, you are going to have to move and let these people through." She broke down in uncontrollable tears of despair and finally relented.

The barbed wire fence of our private property line was cut, and the giant machines began moving forward, slowly slashing a wide swath and destroying everything in their path. They proceeded, in what was a bitter humiliation, directly through the middle of the pine tree field, knocking down the trees that had grown so tall. It was crushing to see precious memories being hauled away.

Honeysuckle, persimmon trees, and blackberry vines in the path of destruction crumbled as the monsters pressed forward without mercy, cutting another fence line as they entered the largest of the meadows. The acres of tall fescue grass, with stems and seed heads almost four feet tall, waved back and forth in the gentle wind as the blades of the machines stripped the ground leaving the landscape barren and bleak

The call of the bobwhite could no longer be heard. Doves, rabbits, and squirrels fled in terror as the invaders' unrelenting assault continued. Fox, deer, raccoon, and opossum all ran for their life as the agonizing roar of the giant earthmovers echoed though the surrounding woods and creek beds. Thick smoke bellowed from the machines, and the smell of diesel fuel filled the air.

On this day, even Mama's yellow butterfly was nowhere to be found. The small middle pond, which had been a watering hole for cattle and other thirsty creatures for so many years was obliterated in seconds. And then, in one final act of treachery, the machines plowed through the shady lane, cutting it in half, before exiting the property, taking the heart of a family with them.

Our parents had nurtured this land for years while protecting it from trespassers and thieves. They had intended to live here for the rest of their lives and then pass on the treasure to succeeding generations. Now, they would stand as an outsider surveying the damage that had been done to what once was their land.

They would now be the trespassers on the land that had just been seized by the state. The property had been cut almost in half. There was no way to get to the fifteen acres, which remained on the other side of the swath that had just been cut without crossing over the land, which was now controlled by the highway department.

It was all gone in what seemed like just minutes. The state could seize the private property against the will of the private property owner under a law, which gives the state the right of imminent domain to take private property that will be used for the benefit of the public.

The government, through the right of imminent domain, had taken the property, along with the property of countless others, to build Interstate 24—a highway with a western terminus in Southern Illinois and an eastern terminus in Chattanooga, Tennessee. The path of the highway took it across the Ohio River through Paducah continuing with a northwest to southeast orientation. This would be the first exit off the interstate heading south after crossing the Ohio River from Illinois into Kentucky. This doorway to Dixie was designated as exit number 3.

The highway would split our property into two almost equal halves and leave both halves completely landlocked. A diamond-shaped interchange with entrance and exit ramps for the highway was also to be built connecting with Old Cairo Road. The highway exit ramp fence would run adjacent to Old Cairo Road and across the entire front of our property.

An access road was constructed for the landlocked back half of our property. We would have to travel on three different roads to access the property. Anyone could drive down that road onto our property, and we had no way to monitor who was trespassing or what they were doing. We would catch people engaged in all sorts of activities including illegal fishing. It quickly became known as a secluded place to go parking as well.

A significant part of our front yard would also be taken for the highway using the imminent domain law. The U-shaped gravel driveway entrance to the office and house was completely cut off. This would potentially have very damaging effects on Daddy's business and the family's livelihood. An access road for ingress and egress into the property would be built by the highway department. The entrance would be controlled by the highway department and shared with adjacent property owners.

Our home and business would be the closest residence and business to the interstate. The once serene and quite evenings would be shattered by all of the noise that accompanies a major interstate highway. The once private and secluded property would now be completely exposed on all sides to all who traveled the interstate.

Though the interstate had cut the property in half and significantly altered the front of the property, our home remained. We would stay, at least for now, knowing that it was much less safe, and that the once large magnificent farm and surrounding community was completely and forever changed.

The state had offered people whose land they had taken what they considered the fair market value for their homes and property. Mother and Daddy, along with several other families, refused the offers and were taken to court by the state in order to enforce the right of imminent domain.

The neighborhood had already mostly disappeared in preparation for this day. Houses had been torn down or moved as families were forced to find a new place to live. Olivet Baptist Church abandoned its building and built a new church building on Highway 60.

The local grocery store was gone, and all that was left was what seemed like an empty landscape desolate and abandoned.

The old, wooden red barn with the tin roof was gone. Gone too was the field of dreams in front of the barn where countless games of softball, football, and basketball had been played over the years with friends and neighbors. Several of the tall old oak trees closest to the road had been lost to the progress of the highway.

The barbed wire fence lines, filled with shade trees, which had separated the pastures, had been lost to the bulldozers. Our nearest neighbors on either side, like the neighbors across the road, had moved away, and their houses had been moved or torn down. Olivet Church Road had been rerouted to connect with Old Cairo Road about half of a mile west of its original location.

Over the ensuing months, numerous truckloads of gravel and dirt would be hauled to the site to build up the bed of the interstate to almost twenty feet. Then, while work was being completed further south from the Ohio River, the highway would sit for months unpaved for several miles.

This provided a great place to walk, explore, and ride the minibike and bicycles. For the first time, we could easily walk or ride the almost four miles to the Ohio River. Since there was no traffic, we would walk out onto the newly completed Ohio River Bridge and could even make the very long walk all the way across the new bridge to Illinois.

It was quite an experience to walk out onto the long and narrow catwalk underneath the new bridge. The wide and deep river would be swiftly flowing, and the catwalk would sway and bounce with the wind making it difficult to stand at times. The railing on the side of the catwalk was not very high and the possibility of accidentally falling into the river was real. We, nevertheless, greatly enjoyed the brief opportunity to have the interstate and bridge all to ourselves.

One could easily walk under the interstate, from one side of our property to the other, through the large circular concrete drainage culvert that ran under Interstate 24. And since there was no traffic at this time, it was easy to climb the fence and walk across the four lanes of the interstate to get to the large pond, woods, and meadow on the back part of our property.

Soon a new regional mall would be built at the next exit south of exit number 3 on what was once Mr. Potter's peach orchard. The new mall would begin a rapid development of businesses along Highway 60 near the interchange. This would impact Paducah's downtown area as businesses moved out of downtown to relocate near the new mall.

The late nineteen seventies and eighties saw the decline of the downtown area and surrounding neighborhoods as homes deteriorated and crime increased. But Paducah would begin to rebound in the nineties as the National Quilt Museum, the world's largest and most prestigious museum devoted to quilts and fiber art, was built in 1991 in the downtown area.

Just west of downtown lies the Lower Town Fine Arts District, a neighborhood of old homes that have been converted into artist's studios. The vibrant Arts and Small Business District is now listed on the

National Register of Historic Places. This, along with the Lower Town Arts and Music festival, the Dogwood festival, and the Paducah Summer Festival, draws thousands of visitors, including many international visitors, to Paducah each year. Paducah is now one of America's best small-town comeback stories.

The area around exit number 3 did not develop as fast or in the same manner as the Highway 60 area. For years, there was one small convenience store on one side of the interstate and a truck stop on the other side.

It was thought that though our parents' farm had been devastated by the building of the interstate, the land would actually increase in value because it was adjacent to the exit. However, although the area around the interchange was quickly annexed by the city, services such as water and sewer were not provided to that side of the interstate.

This, and the fact that the property was landlocked, greatly hampered the ability to develop or sell the land. And these acres of land that once were loved so deeply by our parents would become the source of great trepidation for the remaining years of their lives.

The probability that corruption was a major factor in the decision to extend the exit fence made the outcome even more difficult for them to accept. The original plans for the off ramp had the fence running adjacent to Old Cairo Road but stopping before completely cutting off our driveway.

That initial plan was mysteriously revised, and the final plan had the fence extending past the driveway and all the way to the end of the property line. One of the engineers involved with the design of the interchange project purchased land next to ours knowing that his would be the first property with unobstructed access. This made his new purchase much more valuable for commercial use.

Mother and Daddy had contacted local, state, and national officials to review the events and circumstances surrounding the unexplained extension of the fence. There seemed to be more than enough evidence of collusion and fraud to warrant further investigation. The case reached the ears of several high-ranking officials including Governors Wendell Ford and Julian Carroll who did come to physically inspect the situation. In the end, however, nothing was done to change the situation. At one point, Mother climbed a tree and, for several hours over several days, held a large sign that read "Don't Fence Me In."

Today, remnants of those pine trees that my parents planted so long ago still stand tall on either side of the interstate. They still have a story to tell to the people who drive by on Interstate 24. "Here once stood a proud forest planted with love, which was destroyed in minutes, shattering the dreams of those who had no power against the authorities to prevent it."

In the late 1980s, the four children formed the BEKA Group Inc., a subchapter S family corporation, with the land at exit number 3 as partial collateral. The acronym BEKA is formed from the first letter of each of our middle names.

Three convenience stores were purchased in the Nashville area, and a fourth brand-new store was opened in Hopkinsville, Kentucky. Ed served as president of the corporation and ran the business operations. After a while, Tom moved his family to Nashville and served as the business manager.

Voters in Kentucky had approved a lottery, which would begin on the day of the grand opening of the Kentucky store. Our store was selected as one to be visited by Wallace Wilkinson, the governor of Kentucky, as he toured the state to promote the new Kentucky lottery. The story was to make national news headlines as CNN was set to cover the governor's visit, but an earthquake in California, during the World Series, preempted coverage of the event. The grand opening was a huge success as was the visit by the governor and plans for further expansion was underway.

I think the best part of that experience was my young family moving to Nashville where we could be closer to Ed and Laurie and their young family. The stores did very well and the plans for expansion were underway when an unscrupulous realtor deceitfully undercut the lease on two of the stores. This created a downward spiral and the company was eventually dissolved.

ANOTHER SHOCKING LOSS: EVERYTHING

Mother's flowers were in full and glorious bloom in early spring of 1971, as we read an article in the newspaper about a house not far from ours that had burned completely to the ground. No one was home at the time, and no one was injured. But it was particularly sad to hear of tragedy affecting a family who lived in our community.

At the end of April 1971, Mildred, Ed, Carl, and I went to Oxford, Mississippi, to visit Billy, Gayle, Lara, and Karen for the weekend. Carl was a friend of the family who had become friends with Billy and Gayle when Billy taught at Lone Oak High School. Billy was completing his studies to earn a master's degree at the University of Mississippi.

A good time was had by all, and on Sunday, May 2, we piled in Mildred's Dodge Dart and headed for home. Lara Gayle, who was three years old at the time, went with us to visit for a while. Tax time was over, and Mother and Daddy were winding down from the season and looking forward to Lara's visit.

As we traveled down Olivet Church Road, approaching the house, we noticed a band of smoke rising in the direction we were heading. It got a little quieter in the car, and I believe we all had a little nervous sinking feeling in our stomachs while hoping it was just someone burning wood and leaves.

We pulled up to the stop sign at the intersection of Old Cairo Road, and a member of the Concord Volunteer Fire Department was rerouting traffic away from the direction that we were headed. Dennis was a good friend whom I went to school with, and I asked him what was burning. With a look of sadness on his face, he said, "Tom, it's your house."

As we drove within view, we could see the smoldering ashes of what once was our home and my father's office. It had all burned completely to the ground. Neighbors were gathered in different groups. One of our cars had been pushed away from the house and was out in the front yard halfway to the road.

The fire department was still there finishing their duties and preparing to leave. We were told that something inside had exploded as the fire spread from the house to the office blasting the roof of the office about two feet in the air and knocking one fireman off the roof to the ground. It was an oxygen tank that was stored in the corner of the utility room between the house and office.

We did not see Mother or Daddy. As we got out of the car, our neighbors from across the road came and talked with us. We asked where Mother and Daddy were. They did not know. No one had seen them. The other car was not there, and we assumed that mother had gone somewhere and would be home soon. It was Sunday afternoon, so they would have already been home from church. It would not have been uncommon for Daddy to be upstairs or on the couch taking a nap this time of the afternoon. What if he was in the house and did not make it out?

The neighbors invited us to their house, and we sat mostly in shock in their living room trying to make sense of it all. Not much was said, and it seemed like forever until finally, someone said that Mother and Daddy had just driven up. They were together.

It is impossible to explain the sense of relief when the Chrysler Imperial drove up on May 2, 1971, and Daddy was in the car with Mother. Nor will we ever forget them getting out of the car and for the first few moments standing there stunned, absolutely stunned. No tears. No words, just disbelief. They left a lifetime of hard work and returned to find keepsakes, pictures, treasures, and nearly every material possession gone. We are not sure that either one of them ever fully recovered.

They stood there stunned as they looked at their entire lives and business completely gone before my mom started crying. At least they were okay. They had gone to a restaurant near Kentucky Lake to eat dinner, something they would have never done during tax time. But that was over now.

Our family had lost everything except the clothes we were wearing and what was in the cars. The business with all the information and stored files of clients was gone. The neighbors had pushed the car away from the house when they saw the flames but were unable to save anything. They did go in the backyard and rescue the dog, Heidi, who was chained near the dog house.

I stood silently with Daddy in the driveway as he quietly surveyed the scene. A neighbor walked over and silently stood by Daddy. The neighbor reached his hand toward Dad as if to shake it, and Daddy hesitated and then reached out his hand to accept the money that he was being offered. That moment changed me. For the first time, I saw my dad, a proud and generous man, a man who was always there for others, left with nothing, knowing it was okay to accept the kindness of friends.

Those days changed all of us. In just a few short months, my parents had lost their land through the process of imminent domain. The land that was left was separated by an interstate highway, and the landscape was unrecognizable. Now they had lost their office, home, and earthly possessions.

The tall, proud oak trees and the beautiful flower gardens, now in full bloom, were all that remained of what once was a little piece of paradise in which so much of my parents' lives had been invested. They did have insurance on the home and office, which provided for temporary living quarters and helped with the financial burdens of starting over. But insurance cannot replace the most treasured possessions that have accumulated over the years.

We stayed at a hotel for a couple of weeks before temporary housing could be moved to the concrete slab that had served as the foundation for the office. Then they began the process of building a new office and finding a place to live.

The house and office burned exactly one month before my high school graduation. I dressed for some of the graduation events in a hotel room, and Ed finished his sixth grade year. Mildred had moved back home, and she lost everything she had as well. Billy lost some valuable possessions that were stored in the attic.

Ours was the third house in the path of the highway that mysteriously burned when no one was home within about three weeks of each other. I believe they had all been holdouts that did not want to sell or move and their homes completely burned to the ground. No one was home or injured, and though the suspicion of intentional destruction by arson seemed obvious, it was never proven. I don't know if it was seriously investigated.

Baseball once again brought the family together and helped in the healing process. Daddy managed, and I coached Ed's little league baseball team. Mother kept score at the games. It was the only thing that remained familiar and constant in a world that had seemingly been turned upside down.

The search for a new place to live ended after several weeks when they purchased a very small house and twenty-seven acres not far from where the old house was located. It too had secluded pastures and a creek that ran the length of the property. They moved in to what was essentially a two-bedroom home, with three children and very little space for possessions. Of course, we did not have very many possessions.

Ed and I shared a bedroom, and Mildred occupied a bedroom. Mother made a third bedroom in the family room area. It was a small house in a secluded location, but it was home, and after all that had happened, we were all still together.

Our parents believed that they would be able to quickly build a new house in the area across from the driveway. But plans were delayed, and finances were tight. Six years later, after Mildred was married and just after I moved back home to begin dialysis, we moved into the new house.

Billy earned his master's degree from the University of Mississippi and accepted a job teaching mathematics at Meridian Junior College in Meridian, Mississippi, where he and Gayle would raise their family and establish roots over the next thirty-three years. The house in Paducah was too small to house many visitors, so everyone would usually travel to Billy and Gayle's home to celebrate Christmas and for other occasions.

EXIT NUMBER 3

The desolation was complete. The only evidence of what once was a loving home and farm were the dogwoods, azaleas, pine trees, and other shrubbery that now seemed so alone and out of place. They appeared across what was left of the yard and on either side of and in front of the concrete slab that once supported the office.

And then one morning while Mother was driving by, she noticed that the azaleas and roses were gone. In horror, she pulled into the old driveway and realized that someone had stolen many of the azalea bushes, rose bushes, and some of the other plants and shrubs. Once again, devastated, she broke down in tears wondering who could possibly do such a cruel and malicious thing. The only earthly possessions she had left from a lifetime of work and dreams had now been ripped away and taken from her.

She was inconsolable. But within a few hours, someone called and said that he had written down the license number of the truck used to haul away the flowers. The man who had dug up and hauled away the treasure lived up near Kentucky Lake and was one of my father's clients. They knew him. They jumped in the car and headed toward his house.

Sure enough, when they approached his secluded property, the azaleas and other plants that had been stolen were clearly visible. He had already replanted a few, but most were sitting around various parts of his property. Mother and Daddy confronted him, and he readily admitted that he was the one who had taken the azaleas. He apologized and offered to return everything he had taken.

Our parents did not press charges against the thief. They simply allowed him to return the plants to the new home location, which he did that very day. The azaleas were planted across the driveway, in a field adjacent to the one lane road that ran in front of the property and would someday be the location of a new home. Some were planted on a slope of a hill in front of the barn overlooking that field and near a large pecan tree that bore lots of pecans in season.

The blueberry bushes were brought over from the old home site and planted on the slope of the hill. And some of the other plants that had not been stolen were also relocated to the new farm. After all of the tragedy and treachery of the recent past, dealing with the highway department, imminent domain, the house burning, and the azaleas stolen, our parents were finally settling in to a new future.

They had started over so many times, moving and establishing new roots with new dreams while caring for their children in good times and bad. But they were much older now, and the unplanned and unexpected changes would take their toll. For twenty years, they had poured their hopes and dreams into the farm that was now on exit number 3, and now it was all gone. But they had bounced back before, and it was time to do it again.

The old home site was now completely landlocked on both sides of the interstate, deserted and desolate with no buildings on the grounds. The only access to the property was by a one lane gravel access road in the front and an even longer access road for the back of the property.

That was not the end of the problems at exit number 3. The entrance to the access road off of Old Cairo Road into our property was solely for our use. At least, that is what our parents were told when they extended the fence to the end of our property line, landlocking the property. The engineer, who mysteriously made the change that would extend the fence, had sold the property, and now, as one might expect, a convenience store with gas pumps was built on the land adjacent to ours.

The culvert and entrance, built solely to access our property, was now shared with a prosperous business that generated a lot of traffic. Our mom was going over to visit the property one day and found the turn into our property completely blocked by a large truck. This had serious and severe consequences. There were still twenty-seven acres remaining on this side of the interstate, and the value of the property was expected to increase over time since it was the first exit into Kentucky. But the property would be worthless if there was no clear and unobstructed access to the land.

This is what our parents had feared when all of the intrigue over the length of the fence was being played out. The battle to save their land was not over. Mother would drive her car to the location and sit in her parked car at the entrance so that no one could block access to our land. This, of course, was not a solution to the problem but served to make the point that the betrayal had been consummated, her land was not protected, and corrective action was needed immediately.

If her land were to be developed, with new businesses someday, she wanted it to be something attractive for the area and beneficial to the local community. She resisted all offers to buy the property from people who were planning to build a truck stop. She believed that the full property should be developed and that a truck stop was inappropriate for the community.

A couple of years earlier, when Mom and Dad had realized that nothing could be done to prevent the interstate from its route through our property, they knew that the business would have to be moved to a new location that would have less interference from interstate traffic and noise. They also realized that, someday, they would probably have to move from their house. Even though the interstate did not destroy the house, the area would now be developed for commercial use. All of the closest neighbors had already moved or were making plans to move.

They purchased property, about one and one-half acres, on US Highway 60 about one mile from our current home and office. This would be a good location to build a new office. The area would develop quickly after the interstate was complete. The property had an undeveloped lot that could be cleared to build an office building. It also had an old house occupied by the owner. They believed that they could someday sell the house or, if necessary, relocate to the house, which would be next to the new office building.

The owner of the house, Charlie Brown, was an old friend, and together, they completed an agreement that he would have the right to live in the house for the rest of his life. A new office building would be built on the adjacent lot, when possible, and Mother and Daddy would receive possession of the house upon Mr. Brown's death.

The summer after our home burned, the lot on Highway 60 was cleared and prepared so that a new office building could be built. Bulldozers knocked down the taller trees and pushed them into piles. I worked on that lot quite a bit that summer, clearing the thick overgrown brush, cutting wood with chain saws, and burning the piles of timber and brush.

Our blue Ford 2000 tractor, along with the implements, was in the barn when our house burned and survived the fire. Daddy and I used it quite a bit in the lot preparation. We put thousands of hours of useful service on that tractor over the years at both our old Exit 3 farm and at the new home place on Stanley Road. Its sentimental value increased with each passing year. Mother gained a love for that tractor as much as anyone and could sometimes be seen driving it down the roads to the back pond and then back again to Stanley Road.

After mom died, and her children had no place for the tractor, we sold it to our parents dear friends Jimmy and Bobbie Jean Edwards. They were the only ones our mom would have wanted to have the tractor. They still use it today.

The lot on Highway 60 was finally cleared and the new office completed before the start of the next tax season. People quickly learned of the new office location, and, much to our parents relief, business actually increased at the new location.

Within a couple of years, Mr. Brown's health began to fail, and he was moved to a nursing home, leaving the house unoccupied. He had no one to watch over his home and possessions. Mother visited him in the nursing home, assisted him as best she could, and took him things that he requested from the house.

We woke one morning to the news that Mr. Brown's house had burned to the ground the night before, and there was nothing left. It seemed inconceivable that something like this could happen again! An investigation determined that arson had been the cause of the fire.

When Daddy was nearing retirement age, he asked if any of the children would return to or stay in Paducah and take over the business. He had formed Cooper Enterprises Inc. to incorporate his current business and handle any future opportunities that may occur. After much discussion and consideration, it was decided that he would sell the business upon retirement.

Daddy sold his business and the building to the brother of the governor of Kentucky. He worked with the new owner for the first year to help clients adjust. He kept some clients as his own and continued to prepare their accounting and tax requirements from home.

The land at exit number 3 remained vacant. Offers to buy the property were all refused. The next exit south was quickly developed as the primary exit for the area. A new mall was built in what was once a peach orchard. Restaurants and hotels opened, and improvements were made to the roads and infrastructure. The value of the land at exit 3 never significantly increased, and any serious offers to develop the property were never received.

About three months after the house burned and when Mom was fifty years old, she returned to college taking evening classes at Paducah Community College (PCC). That was also my first semester of college at PCC. We had many of the same teachers that year though I was attending day classes. She had challenged me that she would have a better grade point average than I would. That helped to increase my focus. It was a wonderful experience to have the same teachers in the same school as my mom. We both did very well, and I believe we finished with the same grades. Ed and Karen would later also have a few classes with those same teachers.

Mrs. Price, who taught English literature at PCC, and her husband coordinated group tours each summer usually by bus to locations throughout the United States, Canada, and Mexico. Mother and Ed went on the tours several summers and always enjoyed the adventure immensely.

Mother's spirit was one of adventure and exploration. She enjoyed travel, learning, and discovery. These traits were instinctive in her children as well. Both Billy and Mildred have traveled extensively stateside and overseas for work and pleasure. There are not too many places in the states that Ed has not seen. My exploration has been more restrained, though I have been to almost all of the states. I learned from an early age that I should not place myself in circumstances that were beyond my control because of health issues.

STORMS OF LIFE

> Therefore whoever hears these sayings of Mine, and does them, I will liken him to a wise man who built his house on the rock: and the rain descended, the floods came, and the winds blew and beat on that house; and it did not fall, for it was founded on the rock.
>
> —Matthew 7:24–25
> (New King James Version)

We had lost our house to fire and lost the farm to the interstate highway, but the foundation of faith, which had been built on the rock of Christ, though battered and bruised, did not fall. In fact, it was at its greatest strength when faced with adversity.

Our parents were not overtly religious and did not wear their faith on their sleeves. Much like all of us, they were not perfect. Like many people of the greatest generation, their convictions were expressed more in their actions, and the way they lived their lives spoke volumes. They gave their children a foundation of faith that would be indispensable in the years to come.

Faith has always been important in our family. It is an important part of the healing process for the human body both physically and emotionally. And there is no doubt, for me, that every breath I take is a unique and special gift from God. I have known this for a long time and hope that it is never taken for granted. The four of us grew up in a home with parents who valued the Bible and honored men and women of faith.

I can remember a few times, when I was very young, my mom sat in front of the television and asked me to watch Oral Roberts give his message on faith and then pray for the sick in the television audience. Roberts was nationally known and respected for his healing ministry and appeared on national television quite often back then. His prayer of faith, and her faith that his prayer would be answered, was an encouragement to me.

One day, she told me to get in the car because we were going to see someone. It turned out to be a pastor who was known for praying for the sick as a type of faith healer. He lived in a nearby town and had been recommended to my mom by a trusted friend. He did lay hands on me and pray for healing, and I slowly began to understand the critical role that faith plays as part of the healing process of the physical human body.

Each of our parents' children would, in due course, accept salvation and be baptized into the faith. Over the years, and at different times, we, along with our spouses, supported various churches in a manner of ways. We would learn about servant leadership from cleaning the church facilities, teaching Sunday school, leading a youth group, or serving on a committee. Mildred and Rusty have ministered to countless thousands in cities across the country and around the world.

I was christened as an infant at Fountain Avenue Methodist Church in Paducah. Our family later attended Palestine Methodist, and our parents helped to form a new Methodist church in the Concord Community.

The new congregation of Concord Methodist met in the adjacent elementary school while the church was being built. Years later, we also attended Broadway United Methodist in downtown Paducah.

Several of the pastors at Concord and Broadway stand out in my memory as much or more than the teachers in school. Brother Tate made a lasting impression when he complimented the red bow tie my mother had dressed me in one Sunday. Several pastors and their wives were friends of the family for many years. Among them were the Reverends G.E. Clayton and Bill Riley who performed the service at our father's funeral. Brother Russell and his wife, Grace, were long-time friends of my parents and he, along with Rusty, performed the services at our mom's funeral. Other pastors left positive impression for their kindness and examples of faith.

Mother would occasionally be asked to play the piano at an evening service at Concord when the primary piano player was unavailable. She loved to play but was uneasy with this task because she was mostly self-taught and not as proficient at playing as she would have preferred. Mildred took piano lessons when she was young and also gained a love for playing the piano. I would be asked to serve as an usher on a regular basis at Concord and Broadway when in high school and college.

I attended Paducah Community College for two years after high school and then transferred to Western Kentucky University in Bowling Green, Kentucky. Shortly after arriving on campus, I started a Bible study and prayer group in my dorm room. The small group that evolved shared their faith around campus, handed out tracts, and fostered relationships with students, faculty, and staff. The group sought and received recognition by the university as a student organization.

The Christian music group Lamb was touring in the area the next spring, and we booked them for a concert on campus. I met with administrators of the university and members of the Student Government Association (SGA) to seek permission for Lamb to perform in a large auditorium on campus. The SGA provided partial funding and sponsorship for the concert on campus, and our group hosted the event. Radio and newspapers advertised the event. Fliers were posted all over campus. The result was the largest crowd to ever attend a concert sponsored by the SGA at that time.

During my sophomore year of college in Paducah, I attended meetings of the newly organized Maranatha Christian Center. The Paducah church featured a number of well-known Christian artists as guests. Barry McGuire along with the Second Chapter of Acts performed in concert at the Maranatha Center in Paducah on October 29, 1974. Keith Green, Honeytree, John Michael Talbot, Terry Talbot, and Don Francisco were among the many other notables to perform in Paducah and at other ministry locations.

Dozens of prominent men and women would serve as guest instructors at Maranatha Leadership Training Conferences. Included among the many speakers over the years were Winkie Pratney, Pat Boone, Rosey Grier, the Hon. John B. Conlan, Kenneth Hagin, Pat

Robertson, Dr. Chuck Flynn, Charles Schmitt, and Kenneth Copeland.

The sheer number and quality of prominent Christian speakers and musicians who regularly appeared in a small town such as Paducah was unprecedented. And the education was priceless. They each had a part in the development of faith and character in the young believers who attended those events.

Within a few months of its opening, Maranatha was expanding its ministry to college students at universities throughout the region. Soon after the Lamb concert at Western, the Maranatha leadership decided to open a new campus ministry at WKU.

A new Bible study was formed at the Downing Student Center led by a staff member from Paducah. Before long, a former fraternity house on Chestnut Street (fraternity row) became available, and Maranatha secured a lease. The house was in an excellent location; however, it was in poor condition and much work needed to be done. The house was restored with much assistance from student and community volunteers and volunteers from the Paducah fellowship.

Bowling Green High School opened up its doors for an outreach, which aided in announcing the opening of the center. Assemblies, featuring the singing group Praise, were covered by Bowling Green's WBKO-TV. These assemblies led into smaller classroom appearances that led to one student being freed from drugs and thirty making individual commitments to Christ. The movie *Son Worshippers* was also shown in the high school.

On opening night, a crowd of two hundred people made their way into the center. The crowds continued throughout opening week with dozens of people receiving the gift of salvation through Christ.

The ministry staff consisted of three full-time staff and five part-time staffers. Regular meetings were scheduled on Monday and Thursday nights at 7:00 p.m. Bible studies on the fundamentals of faith in Jesus were held on Sundays at 7:00 p.m. A men's prayer breakfast was held every Wednesday at 6:00 a.m. A dedicated phone number to be used as a hotline was acquired.

A couple of years later, I became the director of a campus ministry at Morehead State University in Morehead, Kentucky, and part of a ten-member team with ministries at the University of Kentucky and Eastern Kentucky University.

Over the next few months, many of the nationally acclaimed Christian musicians who had performed at the Paducah Church would also perform in concert at the three universities. The movies *Cross and the Switchblade*, *Sports Odyssey*, *What's up Josh*, *Gospel Road*, and *Son Worshippers* were featured at MSU.

RISE AND SHINE AND GIVE GOD THE GLORY

The months I spent on dialysis and recovering from the transplant would provide some of the most treasured times of Bible study and meditation. I am convinced that laughter is good medicine. I am also convinced that faith can play a significant role in the process of physical, psychological, and spiritual healing.

I underlined and highlighted many scripture verses as I read through the Bible. There is no greater source of comfort and hope than what is contained within the pages of that book. I was inspired, in part, by the life of Christy Mathewson, one of the greatest baseball pitchers of all time.

Cristy has his place in the baseball hall of fame in Cooperstown, New York. The floors of that facility contain treasured artifacts and relics of the game. There is a bat used by Babe Ruth and a glove worn by Lou Gehrig. Shoes and jerseys worn by other great players line the walls of the baseball cathedral.

In one glass case, an exhibit contains an artifact unlike any other. It is an old, worn Bible, spread open, with all the evidence of many years of constant use. The book itself and the explanatory card with it are testimony to the character of its former owner. The card states: "This Bible belonged to and was used by Christy Mathewson."

I hope someday my Bible may be as used as his was. I could write volumes about the lessons of life learned from the scripture. The following are some that may help each of us as we struggle with life's storms. This is by no means an exhaustive list. It is simply a few of the many verses that offered encouragement during a difficult time.

> A merry heart does good, like medicine, But a broken spirit dries the bones. (Proverbs 17:22)

He has shown you, O man, what is good; And what does the LORD require of you But to do justly, To love mercy, And to walk humbly with your God? (Micah 6: 8)

Yet in all these things we are more than conquerors through Him who loved us. For I am persuaded that neither death nor life, nor angels nor principalities nor powers, nor things present nor things to come, nor height nor depth, nor any other created thing shall be able to separate us from the love of God which is in Christ Jesus our Lord. (Romans 8: 37–39)

But it is good for me to draw near to God; I have put my trust in the Lord GOD, That I may declare all Your works. (Psalms 73:28)

"My grace is sufficient for you, for My strength is made perfect in weakness." Therefore most gladly I will rather boast in my infirmities, that the power of Christ may rest upon me. Therefore, I take pleasure in infirmities, in reproaches, in needs, in persecutions, in distresses, for Christ's sake. For when I am weak, then I am strong. (2 Corinthians 12:9–10)

"For My thoughts are not your thoughts, Nor are your ways My ways," says the LORD. "For as the heavens are higher than the earth, So are My ways higher than your ways, And My thoughts than your thoughts." (Isaiah 55:8)

"They sow the wind, and reap the whirlwind." (Hosea 8:7)

> Jesus answered him, "The first of all the commandments is: 'Hear, O Israel, the LORD our God, the LORD is one. And you shall love the LORD your God with all your heart, with all your soul, with all your mind, and with all your strength.' This is the first commandment. And the second, like it, is this: 'You shall love your neighbor as yourself.' There is no other commandment greater than these." (Mark 12:30)

> Finally, brethren, whatever things are true, whatever things are noble, whatever things are just, whatever things are pure, whatever things are lovely, whatever things are of good report, if there is any virtue and if there is anything praiseworthy-meditate on these things. (Philippians 4:8)

> But I am like a green olive tree in the house of God; I trust in the mercy of God forever and ever. I will praise You forever, Because You have done it; And in the presence of Your saints I will wait on Your name, for it is good. (Psalms 52:8)

I believe that it is important to begin to serve God when you are young. Don't wait until you are out of college or married or old. The greatest joy comes from a lifelong walk of faith.

Though I did not know it at the time, the symptoms of kidney failure and heart failure would soon surface in my life. New storms would rise, and once again, things would dramatically change for our family.

STANDING ON THE PROMISES

At age twenty-four, my physical strength and stamina began to fail. I did not realize, at first, how sick I had become. But I knew that I needed to go home to the place where I knew there would be help. I was really sick this time: feet swollen, could barely breathe, barely walk. I suspected that there would probably be no leaving home to get on with my life this time. And so it was.

I had worked for my father, in his accounting practice, for a year after graduating college. After that year, a crucial decision had to be made. I was chosen to be a coleader of a team that would begin a new campus ministry on a campus six hours from home. I accepted that assignment and relocated to Morehead, Kentucky, about one hour east of Lexington.

Within three or four months of the move, I began to feel very sick in a way that I had never experienced. As codirector of a college campus Christian ministry at Morehead State University, I did not want to let down or leave my team. We were already seeing great results toward building a successful long-term ministry. As usual, I did not want people to know how bad I was feeling, but they clearly knew something was not right.

The fear of letting my friends and coworkers down was distressing. I did confide with a few people about my lack of energy and rapidly decreasing stamina, swelling of the ankles, and inability to concentrate or focus on details.

As my strength began to fail, I found myself conflicted between faith and the immediacy of the issues of life. I was asked to give an inspirational sermon in Lexington, Kentucky, to a group of college students from three different area universities. I prepared as best I could, and when the evening came, our team traveled to Lexington and onto the auditorium. As the time approached for me to take my place on the stage and present the message, my strength completely failed. I was embarrassed and ashamed as they encouraged me to give it a shot, and I had to confess that I could not.

At a very important moment, I felt like I had let my team down. I had let the audience down and had probably let God down. After trying for so many years to overcome and work through so many health concerns, when I was finally put in a major spotlight, I failed because of disease. But I was too sick to explain much. Fortunately, our team was headed back home to Paducah for a weeklong conference at the church headquarters. I knew that I would probably not be returning.

Once home for a day, my father, realizing how sick I was, carried me to the car and into the emergency room of the hospital. He was there when the doctor, a longtime friend of his, came to my hospital bedside. "You have heart failure, kidney failure, and other organs are shutting down. We may be able to save your life for now, but you will need dialysis for the rest of your life. Maybe a kidney transplant if you qualify later down the road."

The irony in this is not the diagnosis. I had dealt with serious medical issues for as long as I could remember. But my father was in the room with me to hear this. He had always been too busy at work or taking care of the necessities of family life to be with me at a doctor event, unless the doctor had come by the house to treat me. It was usually my mom who took care of everything medical. *Did this mean that somehow this was much more serious this time?* In my heart, I knew it was.

During the two-week hospital stay, vital signs were stabilized and discussions about dialysis began. Although I did not need to begin dialysis immediately, it would only be a matter of weeks before it became necessary to save my life. Dialysis is a treatment that does some of the things done by healthy kidneys. You need dialysis when you develop end-stage kidney failure. This is usually by the time one loses 85 to 90 percent of kidney function. The process removes waste, salt, and excess water from the body, helps regulate blood pressure, and helps keep safe levels of certain chemicals in the blood.

I was taken to surgery for a minor procedure that would create an internal arteriovenous (AV) fistula in my left arm. This procedure is a surgical connection of an artery and a vein. Once mature, it is where they insert the needles for the blood to flow to the dialysis machine. It can take three months or so from "creation" until it is ready to use.

An external shunt would be necessary if the internal fistula was not ready for use. The access point for the dialysis needles is always a continuing concern. They are fairly large needles and need to be inserted where blood flow will be best. Over time, access points can weaken, and a different area of the body would be used for access. Long-term dialysis patients, and those with weaker veins, may have used several different access points over time.

The doctor also discussed the two types of dialysis, hemodialysis and peritoneal dialysis. At the time, peritoneal dialysis was done but was not common. I would undergo hemodialysis at the dialysis treatment clinic at Lourdes Hospital in Paducah.

Kidney function may improve with dialysis for some kinds of acute kidney failure. For end-stage kidney failure, however, kidney failure is permanent.

I was placed on a very strict sodium-free diet that limited the amount of protein, daily fluid intake, and food consumption. About three months later, the dialysis treatments began. I stuck to the diet pretty well, only cheating a few times with a cheeseburger and fries at Griff's Burger Bar or similar establishment.

It is not uncommon to lose several pounds of body weight during the procedure. The length of the hemodialysis process depends on several factors. Generally, it is a three- to four-hour process that is needed three times a week. If one stops the treatments for any reason, death will normally occur within days.

Sometimes leg cramps would occur after dialysis as well as dizziness while standing or walking after the treatment was finished. I usually felt better with more stamina after the treatments but also usually needed to rest for a while.

During the process, however, the dietary restrictions were lifted, and one could eat and drink whatever he would like, a small consolation for an otherwise disquieting procedure. The dialysis unit is not usually a place for the squeamish to visit. I was fortunate to have a number of family and friends drop by for a few minutes from time to time to say hello and help pass the time.

Phyllis, a dear friend and nurse at the hospital, would bring books and snacks along with an occasional slice of pizza, along with comforting conversation. She would sometimes bring things for the other people hooked up on the machines as well. Everyone was always happy to see her, and the mood of the room brightened noticeably while she was there. Debbie, another dear friend, would sometimes sit with me and work on her knitting while passing the time. That, too, was a special gift of providing comfort and companionship by a friend.

Dialysis, however, is a treatment to help manage a disease and is not a cure. Likewise, a transplant is a treatment with an indefinite success rate. Since the opportunity to receive a transplant is not guaranteed, dialysis must often be viewed as a permanent routine for the rest of one's life.

Over time, some people tolerate the procedure better than others. Though no one knows for sure how long one can survive on dialysis, it is thought that it is possible for some patients to live a long and healthy life.

As is the case with most diseases, statistics, success rates, and treatment options are discussed almost immediately and can often be confusing or even overwhelming. For patients with chronic kidney disease, the treatment options are few, but the statistics are numerous. Treatment is either dialysis or kidney transplant.

The average success rates of each vary and are different with each patient.

Dr. Jackson, the nephrologist who treated me in Paducah, contacted the renal transplant team in Nashville and scheduled an appointment for me to be seen by Dr. Johnson. I would be evaluated by the transplant team to see if I was eligible for a kidney transplant.

Dr. Johnson served as medical director of the Kidney Transplant Program at Vanderbilt University Medical Center for over twenty-five years. He is founder of the Tennessee Donor Services and has been president of the United Network for Organ Sharing (UNOS), the Association of Organ Procurement Organizations (AOPO), and the Southeastern Organ Procurement Foundation (SEOPF) at various times during his career. He has since retired from his Vanderbilt position and devotes his time to the management of Dialysis Clinic Inc. (DCI).

He is the founding and principal nephrologist of DCI, the nation's largest not-for-profit dialysis care provider dedicated to the care of renal patients. Dr. Johnson's legendary leadership has allowed DCI to commit more than $100 million to research, education, and nonprofit activities such as Camp Okawehna, a weeklong summer experience for children with kidney disease. Dr. Johnson provides the medical direction for Camp Okawehna. Ed has served as a volunteer at Camp Okawehna in recent years.

Extensive testing was completed, and the transplant team established that I was eligible for transplant and for placement on the waiting list to receive a kidney.

I was placed on the list but with low priority so that potential living donors could be screened for compatibility. Ed was considered to be the best potential donor match among family members, and he was only seventeen when dialysis began. He would be tested to see if he were a match when he was eighteen years old. Percentages showed that donor organs from a living relative were a much better match with a greater chance for long-term success of the grafted kidney.

MATCHING SCARS

So at age twenty-four, I had moved back home with my parents and Ed. It was a very comfortable place to get on with the business of healing, and I felt fortunate to be able to have my parents and Ed there providing a sense of normalcy. My mom helped tremendously with food and the dietary restrictions. Ed and I grew even closer, if possible, as we talked late into the nights, watched *The Rockford Files*, *Hawaii Five-O*, *M*A*S*H*, and other television shows together. We watched and played sports when we could and would confide with one another often.

My dad had helped with the insurance, Medicare, financial, and other issues that a young man would find daunting at best. The urgency of the moment and the uncertainty of the future were constant reminders that my life had forever changed.

The winter of 1978 was a particularly snowy one for the Paducah area. At one point, I had to put snow chains on the old Ford Pinto in order to get to and from the hospital for dialysis treatments. I could usually drive myself there and back, but occasionally, Ed or someone else would volunteer to drive if I had not recovered well from the treatment.

After a few months, I got a part-time job at the Ford dealership to help with expenses. Dialysis patients, at that time, were pretty much restricted to the one facility where they receive treatment, making arrangements to travel for an extended period difficult. There were not as many dialysis facilities throughout the country as there are today. I did make arrangements in the summer to transfer treatment to a dialysis facility in Athens, Georgia, where I would visit Mildred for a few weeks. Treatments were coordinated with the dialysis center in Athens without any disruption.

Ed was tested after he turned eighteen enduring a battery of tests to determine if he would be an eligible donor. As mentioned earlier, Ed was a freshman in college when the donation process began. During the examination period, doctors discovered that Ed's left kidney had three arteries, while his right kidney had two. Typically, a kidney has a single artery, and traditionally, the medical team removes the donor's left kidney for transplantation. This raised the stakes for him as a donor, and the transplant was postponed.

Six months later Ed got the call and was told that the team had decided to take his right kidney and make if work if he was willing to take the risk. He told them that there was nothing to think about, and that he was ready to do it.

A transplant date was soon established. Two brothers, who had been so close all of their lives, were now awaiting a date that would bond them together for life in a way that only a few had ever attempted or could possibly imagine.

This was my little brother laying down his life for me, being strong for the both of us when I was most vulnerable. This was a special kind of sacrificial love. This was Ed giving a part of himself to his brother.

How could I possibly allow him to do this? My little brother, whose welfare I have watched over and guarded all his life. And now, I am placing his life at risk. What if something went terribly wrong?

I did not need to be reminded of what a special gift this would be. But my mom lovingly reminded me a few times in a kind and gentle way, and I was so glad that she did. The fact that she and Daddy approved of the transplant and encouraged us to go through with it helped to reassure me that it was the right thing to do.

On Sunday, February 18, 1979, we loaded the cars, and Ed and Mom headed toward Nashville in one car with Daddy and me following in another. After checking in at Vanderbilt, we were placed as the only two in a four-bed ward to prepare for the surgery Tuesday morning.

More tests were done for both of us. The transplant team would visit us as well as counselors of all types. We were told what recovery time to expect after the surgery.

Monday morning, I underwent my last dialysis treatment. I remember thinking and praying that this would be the last one ever for me. I was lying down during this treatment, instead of sitting in a recliner-type chair, and slept through most of the procedure.

Tuesday morning, Mom and Dad were both there early in the morning waiting with Ed and me as they came to get both of us to take us to surgery. Ed and I gave each other a final reassuring glance as they rolled us away to separate areas of the operating room.

One of the decisions that had to be made during the evaluation process was whether or not to remove the two old kidneys. Normally, if this was done, there would be a first surgery a few weeks prior to the transplant to remove the old kidneys.

I had high blood pressure while on dialysis and needed medication to control it. Because my blood pressure had not been an issue prior to dialysis, it was thought that it would return to normal after the transplant, and they decided not to perform the surgery to remove the old kidneys.

After Ed and I arrived at Vanderbilt for the transplant, we were told that they had decided that they would remove the old kidneys during the transplant. Though not the common practice, it had been done before and the risk was low. Removing the old kidneys would necessitate placing the new kidney in my lower right abdomen instead of the lower back area where the kidneys are normally located. This would extend the length of the surgery, but only minimally.

However, when they were taking the old kidneys out and preparing the new graft area, it was discovered that my appendix was highly inflamed. The appendix was removed along with the old kidneys, and this did lengthen the surgical time.

The doctors later told us that it was a good thing that they had discovered and removed the appendix. It could have ruptured at some point soon after the transplant. If that had happened, when symptoms occurred, I would probably been treated for rejection of the kidney instead of appendicitis and, as a result, could have died.

The doctors had already opened Ed up in the adjacent operating room and now needed to wait before removing his kidney. Vanderbilt is a teaching hospital, and there were a number of students observing the proceedings. Since they had unanticipated extra time after opening Ed, they had the students identify and examine several of Ed's organs while they waited for the other team to finish preparing me.

One of the students later told Ed that examining a living patient's organs in such a manner was an opportunity that most did not have. We acknowledged the humor in her comments with a somewhat nervous laugh. So Ed was not only a living donor that day; he was a living teaching aide as well.

Once they had me ready, they removed Ed's kidney and carried it the few feet to the adjacent room to graft it into my body. It began working immediately after the successful graft was completed.

Ed was taken to the recovery room and then when ready back to our ward. There had been no complications for his surgery. Mother and Daddy were there with him when he woke up.

I remember waking up in ICU with tubes seemingly coming out of every part of my body. I could not speak because of a ventilator but did feel and then see my mom and dad holding my hand as they stood by my bed. It was a glorious sight to behold. They told me that Ed was doing well and that he had no complications. They said that my surgery also had gone well. I squeezed each of their hands as we all tried to hold back the tears.

After a couple of days, I was returned to the ward where Ed was. It is difficult to describe the emotion when I could finally see him again. We had done this together, and he had saved my life. He was still experiencing pretty consistent and uncomfortable pain.

A student nurse was assigned to each of us. It may have been coincidence, but in addition to being very helpful, they were both quite beautiful. And they seemed to become more so each day. I suppose that meant we were getting better. Of course, Ed had a girlfriend, and Laurie visited him after the surgery and talked with him on the phone.

Our mom, however, seemed to think that Meg, the student nurse who was attending me, would be a great addition to our family if I would just make the effort. Moms seem to think it is a simple thing. I never found that to be the case. And I did not feel that I was in the best position to make a good impression or do much about it at the time anyway.

About five to seven days after the transplant, my body began to reject the new kidney. This was not unexpected as it was quite typical at the time, but it was very scary. The transplant team went into action, and in response to the rejection, the physicians "bombed" my system with large amounts of antirejection medication, and I was placed in a hyperbaric oxygen chamber for several hours. Concern subsided after a couple of days of treatment as rejection subsided and my body began to accept the new kidney.

Ed was in the hospital for a week before he was able to return home. I was there seventeen days. Over the next few weeks, the change in my health was remarkable. The twelve-hour a week sessions tied to a dialysis machine with the constant flow of blood in and out of my body through large needles and long tubes was no longer necessary.

Life would slowly return to normal after Ed and I both returned home. I was told to wear a mask when out in public for the first few months to decrease the chance of catching an illness from germs. It was comforting when the doctors told me that the illness and surgery would not prevent me from having children in the future. And my disease is not something that my children could inherit.

There were cautionary statistics provided by the doctors to remind us that transplants are not guaranteed to last forever and that many things could impact the future health of the graft. Yet faith had carried us this far, and faith is what we would rely on for the future.

Plans for the future, uncertain and on hold for most dialysis patients, including me, could now be carefully considered, including the freedom to travel and roam as far and wide as time and finances would allow. Breathing and stamina was much better without the buildup of fluids in my body in-between dialysis sessions.

Spring would arrive and then summer. Eventually, Ed and I could once again be found playing some type of sports and accepting the challenges of pickup basketball games around town. There were times when the competitors discovered they were receiving a stiff challenge from a couple of transplant patients.

Better than any tattoo were the matching zipper scars on our abdomens, from the belly button down, which stood out when we removed our shirts to play on a skins team. We gladly answered the questions of our astonished and curious competitors as they noticed the matching disfigurement.

I unwittingly became very protective of the new graft in my lower right abdomen. When a threat to the area, real or perceived, was attacking, my right arm would instinctively reach up or down in force to deter the threat, much to the surprise of friend or foe and years later even my wife. Though skeptical at first, she lovingly understood when I explained, and she remains cautious to this day of any sudden, unexpected moves to the right abdomen area.

On Christmas night, about ten months after the transplant, the local NBC television affiliate aired a special story about Ed's gift of life. They filmed part of the story at our home and included interviews of Ed, our parents, and me.

Ed would attend classes at the University of Mississippi beginning with the fall semester and transfer to Western Kentucky University in the spring. He and Laurie would later marry and move their family to Nashville where they would raise their three children. They still live in the Nashville area. Ed sometimes volunteers his time to a kidney camp for children suffering from end-stage renal disease. He is often asked to speak at various events where he shares our story.

I was best man at Ed and Laurie's wedding, and Ed was best man when Karen and I were married. Five years after the transplant, Karen and I were married on an icy December day at the church she and her family had attended for years and where her mother was still active. If there was no dialysis or transplant, I would have died, never married, and Karen and I would never have known the glorious joy of the two daughters with which God blessed our lives. Ed's gift has kept on giving through the years.

Ed gave the gift which extended the journey on earth, which was much like being born again—born for the third time in a way. And soon, my two children would teach me a great deal more about why life is such a gift.

I'm not certain that Karen knew what she was getting into by marrying a transplant patient. She knew of the transplant and had even visited me with a group of friends when I was recovering at Vanderbilt. By the time we began dating, however, my life had returned pretty much to normal.

Karen adapted quickly, going to clinic with me and learning about and preparing transplant-friendly foods. We have a wonderful life together though we have been the wanderers of the family. My siblings and her siblings each have deep roots in their communities. We have lived in several states including Colorado, Virginia, Tennessee, and Kentucky.

TRIPLE DEUCES

The old man standing in front of me was serving multiple life sentences for killing and then partially consuming several people. We were surrounded by murderers, mafia kingpins, gang leaders, rapists, and others who, by their actions, had earned their stay at one of the countries toughest prisons.

It was 9:00 p.m., and inmates were milling about the cell block. Some were playing cards, others talking amongst themselves, but almost all paused as they noticed the strangers who had invaded their home this dark and rainy night. Another staff member and I were on a tour of the notorious Lewisburg Maximum Security Federal prison in Lewisburg, Pennsylvania.

We probably would have been mostly ignored by this hardened group except for the fact that the individual I was with was female and quite attractive. Female officers had been working in maximum security federal prisons for several years, but any stranger, especially a female, disrupted the long-established routine and raised suspicion.

You never get used to the sound of the huge grill door clanging shut behind you as you pass through the last checkpoint before your entry into the most secure area of a facility. Your freedom is now restricted, and you can only get out of this prison if you can prove beyond doubt that you are not an inmate. That fact can be sometimes taken for granted at your home duty station where the control room officer knows and can identify you. If you are a stranger visiting a facility, it is a different situation.

Getting into a maximum security prison is not easy for visitors, even bureau staff. Getting out can be even more difficult. The tour ended before the inmates were confined to their cells for the evening and the last inmate count of this day began. We exited the main building of the prison through the portal at the control room, which is the last check point exit at most prisons.

But this was a maximum security prison, and there was one more hurdle to clear before the last gate at the razor wire fence that opened into the parking lot. As a visitor, I stood in a circle drawn on the ground about halfway between the last building and the fence. An officer in the tower waited for the designated amount of time to ensure that I was not under duress and then the signal was given; the last gate opened, and we departed from the facility.

I had the privilege to work in and visit dozens of federal prisons of all security levels during my career with the Federal Bureau of Prisons. For ten years, I was a training specialist and instructor at the bureau's national training center in Aurora, Colorado. This job required occasional travel to various prisons throughout the country to conduct training, implement new financial systems, provide assistance, and conduct reviews or audits.

In Lewisburg, I was conducting a weeklong training class for financial management staff who worked in the northeast region of the bureau.

My career with the bureau began as an accountant at the Federal Correctional Institution (FCI) in Ashland, Kentucky. Ashland is a small city that sits west of the Ohio River, which flows between the borders of Kentucky and West Virginia. Karen and I, along with six-month-old Kelly, moved to Ashland from Paducah where I had taught the previous six years at Draughon's Junior College of Business.

New staff must quickly learn their roles within a prison setting. Safety and security are at the top of the list along with the procedures of responding to emergency situations. Much of this information is learned during the weeklong Intuitional Familiarization training, conducted shortly after starting the job.

There are many more inmates inside a prison than there is staff. Staff does not carry guns inside a prison. All employees regardless of the department where you work must immediately respond to an emergency alarm. One of the methods for activating an alarm was to dial triple deuces (222) on a phone inside the prison.

Employment at a federal prison is conditional on successful completion of a three-week basic training course, which includes firearms, self-defense, various role play scenarios, as well as classroom instruction. The training is conducted at the Federal Law Enforcement Training Academy in Glynco, Georgia. At the time I attended, all federal law enforcement agencies conducted their training at this facility with the exception of the Federal Bureau of Investigation.

The physical demands of the training were quite a challenge for anyone. Almost seven years after the gift of life from my brother, I passed the training with honors and subsequently began my career with the bureau. While I was at Glynco, the space shuttle *Challenger* exploded shortly after launch, killing all seven crew members including the first teacher in space.

A few months after beginning duty at FCI Ashland, I experienced my first spontaneous pneumothorax when my right lung collapsed. The right lung is the one that was damaged and from which the right lobe was removed after I swallowed a bead when I was twenty-one months old. I spent several days in the local hospital recovering. The same lung collapsed again a few months later and then collapsed a third time shortly thereafter.

After the third collapse, it was decided that I should be transferred to Vanderbilt University Medical Center in Nashville for additional evaluation and treatment. We were offered the opportunity to be transferred by helicopter to Vanderbilt, but Karen and I decided that she would drive us there despite the risk. Upon arrival, I was admitted, and the collapsed lung received additional treatment.

The renal transplant team who had performed the transplant years earlier was once again in charge of evaluation and treatment. They referred me to the pulmonary team, additional tests were completed, and chemical pleurodesis with instillation of tetracycline was performed in my right lung in an effort to avoid recurrence. Karen stayed at Ed and Laurie's house in the evenings. I was released from the hospital after a few more days, and we returned to Ashland. We did visit the Grand Ole Opry for the first time before leaving town.

Some of the worst riots in the bureau's history occurred while I was working at the FCI in Ashland. Inmates who had been a part of the 1980 Mariel boatlift seized control of the US penitentiary in Atlanta and the federal prison in Oakdale, Louisiana. The Atlanta riot lasted eleven days and involved more than one hundred hostages. The inmates burned several buildings within the facility. Delta Force soldiers from Fort Bragg, North Carolina, were sent to advise the civilian law enforcement authorities during the standoff.

One of the more notorious inmates in bureau history was released from his confinement, in an isolation cell, by the rioters at the Atlanta prison. Thomas Silverstein had attacked and killed an officer at the United States Penitentiary in Marion, Illinois, in 1983. Hours later, another officer was killed by a different inmate. The two murderers were members of the Aryan Brotherhood, a white-supremacist prison gang. Silverstein was unofficially under a policy of "no human contact" because of his actions and the murder of an officer. This essentially meant that staff would not communicate with him unnecessarily.

The USP at Marion, less than an hour from Paducah, Kentucky, was the most secure federal prison at the time. It had replaced the infamous Alcatraz prison when that facility was closed. USP Marion went into permanent lockdown for the next twenty-three years as a result of these murders. It was later replaced as the most secure federal prison by the United States Penitentiary, Administrative Maximum Facility (ADX) near Florence, Colorado, sometimes called Supermax or the Alcatraz of the Rockies.

After his release by the Cubans, Silverstein's whereabouts on the compound was unknown to bureau officials. This was a matter of great concern because it was feared that he would harm hostages if he had the opportunity. The Cubans were also concerned once they learned of the gravity of the situation and were ultimately able to drug Silverstein and turn him over to federal authorities. The incidents at Atlanta and Oakdale were resolved without any hostages being killed. Only one inmate was killed when an officer fired at him to protect a fellow officer.

Some of my dearest friends are from the bureau family. During my time with the agency, I met some of the finest men and women our country has to offer. Most of us never see the job these dedicated professionals do in keeping us safe twenty-four hours a day every day of the year.

In addition to working at the Central Office and several institutions, I provided training to hundreds of individuals who traveled to the training center from all over the nation and Puerto Rico. The bureau is not perfect and, like any organization, certainly has its share of problems, but the overwhelming majority of employees are men and women of honor, faith, and integrity.

One of the things that set the bureau apart from other federal agencies is the presidential appointment of its directors. The heads of all federal agencies are appointed by each new president. The Bureau of Prisons (BOP) is the only federal agency whose appointed director is a career employee of that agency. The bureau has had only eight directors since its beginning in 1930, and most of those have served their terms at the pleasure of several presidents.

We lived in several different areas of the country when I worked with the BOP, and the BOP family was often our family away from family. I have played in softball leagues on several teams over the years. One of the best memories came while playing for team FPC Millington. The mixed league team was composed of staff from the Federal Prison Camp in Millington, Tennessee. I had recently transferred there from the higher security facility in Memphis.

We often played some very good teams including some composed exclusively of young military personnel from the adjacent naval air station in Millington. Our team was competitive in every game, and we won our share of games. The Warden at FPC Millington was a fairly young, handsome, and energetic man with an athletic build who ran several miles each week to keep in shape. He played the hot corner at third base and was very good at this position.

One beautiful summer evening, the warden was unable to attend the game, and I was asked to play third base. It just happened to be the evening we played the super duper team from the naval air station, which was predominantly special forces types. It was intimidating just sitting in the dugout across the infield from them. They were very confident and ready to destroy all competition and seemed to be taking extra pleasure in playing a team from the prison camp.

Our team did well, and the score was close going into the third inning. From the third base position, I could notice from the conversation and body language that the team now coming to bat had obviously had enough of the close game and seemed to have decided to let loose with a barrage of runs to establish dominance and end any thoughts of losing to a lesser opponent. Their new strategy seemed to be to pick out the weak link in the defense and blast away with balls hit so hard that fielding it would be treacherous if attempted at all. A glance out of the side of my eye let me know that the batter was going to hit it in my direction.

There was a runner on first base with no outs when the batter looked to see my defensive position. Sure enough, he connected, stinging the ball on one hop off the infield as it headed toward left field. I snared the drive with one quick step to my left and threw to second base for a forced out. The next batter crushed a line drive to my right, and I somehow snared it with a backhand reach around ankle high for the second out. They seemed quite upset with me at this point. Instead of choosing a new target, the manager approached the next batter and pointed in my direction as if to say, "Take him out."

The batter was the biggest hunk of muscle and size I had ever encountered in softball competition. As the pitcher released the ball toward home plate, I braced for what was surely a potentially life altering encounter. The line drive was head high to my left, and I nonchalantly reached and snared it for the third out. As our team left the field, the military heroes acknowledged us with a standing ovation and congratulatory comments.

We did not win the game, but I did win the third base position for the rest of the season, an accomplishment I was not sure that I wanted. The warden was not very happy when at the next game, he was asked to play second base. I feared my job may become much more difficult in the coming days with perhaps extra duty on the night shift. But the warden was a gracious man, and a friend, and he took it like the sportsman he was, though obviously not pleased.

A few months later, he would call me at home to let me know that I had been selected for duty as a training instructor at the bureau's national Management and Specialty Training Center in Aurora, Colorado. It was a relief to hear the purpose of his call as I had left work an hour early with permission from my supervisor because I had been without sleep for the most of two days.

The warden had also called me at home the night before at 12:30 to tell me to report to the facility in two hours to open the safe and disburse funds to the Special Operations and Tactics (SORT) team that was traveling to Talladega, Alabama. A riot had broken out at that facility, and our SORT team was one of several called upon to respond.

Karen was in Paducah with Jennifer visiting family, and Kelly stayed with me so she would not miss any first grade classes. I quickly made arrangements with neighbors and carried the still sleeping Kelly to their house before leaving for duty. The mission was accomplished, but I was without sleep for quite some time.

The training center was located in Fort Worth, Texas, when we learned of the transfer. We did not know initially if we would be moving to Texas or Colorado but soon learned that the move would be to

Colorado. I would travel from Colorado to Fort Worth for several months to conduct the training over a three-week period before the training center was moved to Colorado.

SNAPSHOTS OF LIFE

Oh, what a marvelous blessing it is to be the father of two precious little girls. Ed's gift of life allowed me not only to marry my best friend but also to begin to understand why life is such a gift. They grow up so fast, but wow, did we have some fun along the way!

Of course, we had to learn how to be parents on the fly, as they say. I knew far more about parenting before I became one. Then I found out that I knew almost nothing about the practical side of parenting.

Fortunately for us, Kelly and Jennifer knew how to be children. Trusting innocence, with a fascination and delight to experience life, they unwittingly pushed me to work hard and persevere so that we might have as much time as possible together as a family. Hopefully, they might have it better in life than their parents.

Enjoying watching Disney movies without guilt, as a man, was quite a treat. There was Aladin, Fivel, Muppets, and a whole new world of girl things to conquer. Of course, I was happy to pick and choose when I could. I let Mom enjoy the merriment when it was too girlie for me. On occasion, when Mom was not home, I would find myself on the couch with curlers in my hair and makeup expertly applied by, and much to the delight of, the two instigators of the evening's fun.

Kelly, our oldest daughter, was born when we lived in Paducah, and Jennifer was born when we lived in Ashland, Kentucky. Jennifer was actually born in

Huntington, West Virginia, in a hospital, which is about a twenty-five-minute drive from where we lived.

I, however, wishing to note that each of the four of us was born in Kentucky, tell people that Jennifer was born in Kentucky. I intend nothing sinister about this. It's just that, in my mind, we were living in Kentucky when she was born. Jennifer, upon hearing me say this, is relentless in correcting me and adamant to let all listening know that she was born in West Virginia. This long-standing difference of opinion between the two of us seems to have no willing truce offer from either party.

This is not the Hatfield's of West Virginia versus the McCoys of Kentucky, although that feud did occur not too far from Ashland. It's just a friendly difference of interpretation. I now sometimes bring the issue to light just to see if she is listening or perhaps has changed her allegiance. After all, if she ever becomes president, the national shrine will be the house where she lived when she was born, not the hospital in which she was born. But then again, if she is president, I suppose she can make the hospital a national shrine if she chooses to.

Both girls cherish their time growing up in Colorado. We had many family adventures that are now cherished memories. Family road trips would take us to special places throughout the West and very briefly into Mexico. In our packed to the gills blue short base Dodge minivan, we traveled far and wide, stopping at places like Mount Rushmore, the Grand Canyon, and Carlsbad Caverns where we explored and watched the tens of thousands of bats fly out of the bat cave at dusk.

At four corners the girls stretched arms and legs to stand in four states at the same time. Camping trips to the Grand Teton Mountains, Yellowstone National Park, and Rocky Mountain National Park were often short and quick, but blessed with sounds of two curious, funny, and energetic little girls.

The Denver Center for the Performing Arts provided us with some enjoyable cultural adventures. *The Phantom of the Opera* left a memorable impression as did *The Nutcracker*, *The Sound of Music*, *Annie*, and the Colorado Christmas Concert. The girls would dress up in their finest outfits for these events.

Jennifer reminds us of the time we walked out of the Center, after enjoying the *Nutcracker*, to find that one of the vendors was roasting chestnuts on an open fire. We immensely enjoyed the scene of the season's holiday revelers and leisurely strolled around the plaza eating the chestnuts before departing for home.

The girls attended church camp in the summer and participated in church events throughout the year. At home, the sound of two little girls playing with the huge stash of Barbie's seemingly spread all over the house is a priceless memory. Rows of inside tunnels were built in the large finished basement that served as a private playground.

Always on the go, our blue minivan would be packed with kids as we traveled to church and school events, birthday parties, sleepovers, and soccer or basketball practices and games. Kelly played T-ball for a team that I managed when we lived in Bartlett, Tennessee.

Both girls were very good at athletics and enjoyed several sports. They played mostly for recreational league teams though Kelly did play one year of high school softball. I helped with coaching duties when time permitted and assisted with basketball and soccer team duties. Miniature Doberman pinschers, Wolfgang, Glowheart, and Snickers, snuggled with the girls during naps and bedtime and provided endless love, loyalty, and energy. They also provided quite a few litters of puppies. Cats Princess, Tiger Lilly, and Lucky Star tussled with the dogs and protected the territory.

Holy H. Hamster and Minnie provided a glimpse of hamster life. Gold fish, a large rabbit, and a few other animals enjoyed brief but spirited time as family pets. Many hours were spent at zoos in several states as well as Disneyland and SeaWorld in San Diego and Orlando.

In Orlando, Jennifer and Kelly were drenched by Shamu the killer whale as he swam his circles around the giant whale tank much to the dismay of three-year-old Jennifer. Jennifer had dutifully followed her big sister to the front where she stood with her below the rim of the whale tank unaware of what was about to take place. She later reported that she did not mind the drenching by Shamu so much, but the water was very sticky, cold, salty, and smelly.

The Bible says that children are a blessing from God. Certainly, our two have been. They have filled our lives with laughter and joy. We rejoice with them and cry with them when they are hurting. We attempt to teach them about the family that has preceded them, remind them who they are, and help guide them to make decisions that enhance their life as well as others'.

We remind them of the gift of life that their uncle provided and celebrate the anniversary each year. They help remind us of why life is such a gift. Their trusting innocence and sweet smiles melt the heart even when their parents are exasperated.

Karen would sometimes bring the girls to my office at work to visit. I was often in and out of the office, but we always found ways to enjoy the moments. After one such visit, I opened middle drawer of my desk and found an unsigned sticky note on which words of love were written. I opened other drawers to find sticky notes everywhere.

This started a tradition, and after each visit, I would look to find sticky notes on the walls and windows and in the most creative of places. I don't know if they meant to encourage me, or just saw it as fun, but simple things like that are treasures of my memory.

One of the most horrible events that occurred during our time in Denver was the 1999 school shooting at Columbine High School. Though it did not directly affect us, we knew people who had children attending the school. A few days after the shooting, we went to the high school and paid our respects at the numerous memorials set up to honor the victims.

This brought back memories of the shooting at Heath High School that happened in 1997. That shooting killed three and injured five more. My sister and brothers and I, as well as Karen and Laurie, each graduated from Heath. Rusty's dad and a several other realitives also graduated from Heath. We knew many of the families that had children who were killed and injured. Laurie's neice was among the group of students that were fired on. Karen and I and our girls also visited the memorial at Heath.

The trial of Timothy McVeigh, the terrorist who bombed the federal building in Oklahoma City in 1995, was also held in Denver while we were there. A member of our church was a member of the jury for that trial. A few years later, as Chief of Accounting Operations for the Federal Bureau of Prisons, I would approve payment of some of the expenses of McVeigh's 2001 execution from our national programs budget. He was the first federal inmate executed since 1963.

In June of 2001, we moved from Colorado to Fredericksburg, a small town in Virginia near Washington, DC. I would work at the bureau's central office in DC for the next few years. Karen's sister, Jeannie, traveled from her home in Pullman, Washington, to Denver and then helped drive one of our three cars on the trip to Washington. We would reside in temporary quarters for a few weeks before finding our new home in Fredericksburg. Kelly had just received her driving permit and was also able to help drive on the long road trip.

Kelly began her junior year of high school and Jennifer her first year of middle school the day after Labor Day. They both had to tackle the challenge of new schools in an unfamiliar setting and somehow make new friends along the way. On a Tuesday morning of their second week of school, this new neighborhood, and the world, would be forever changed by the events of the next few months.

From my ninth floor office window, I could see the long, thick, black column of smoke rising from the Pentagon into which terrorists had, a moment ago, crashed a plane. Washington, DC, and America were under attack. Our office, like most of the rest of the nation, had been following radio and television coverage of the events unfolding in New York after the second plane crashed into the towers that September 11, 2001.

We were soon alerted that a fourth hijacked plane was believed to be headed for Washington to be, most likely, crashed into the capitol or White House. Those buildings and many others in the city were being evacuated. The three Bureau of Prisons buildings were within the potential impact zone, with the main office located only one block from the capitol. The building where I worked was two blocks from the capitol.

The streets of the city quickly filled with cars, creating a massive traffic jam, as people were either told to leave work and go home or simply believed that they should. I waited with my staff and coworkers for instruction until we received official instructions to leave. One look out of the window, however, at the barely moving traffic told us that we would not be going anywhere very fast. It was just as well. We quickly learned the garage where our fifteen-passenger commuter van, which carried us to work from a commuter lot in Fredericksburg, was parked had been locked down. We could not go anywhere, so we stayed in our offices.

I attempted to call Karen to let her know that I was okay and that I would be home when I could, but cell phone lines and landlines were jammed. Unable to get a call to connect to home, I tried to call Ed's house in Nashville, and sure enough the call went through. Laurie answered the phone, and after we talked, she called Karen.

At about 12:30, the garage was opened, and we piled into the van to head home. By this time, the streets were eerily deserted, and we made our fastest trip back to Fredericksburg slowing only to observe the scene unfolding at the Pentagon as we passed.

Exactly one week after the terrorist attacks on 9-11-2001, anthrax attacks began in the United States. Over the next few weeks, several letters containing anthrax spores were mailed to locations in New York, Florida, and the DC area killing five people and infecting seventeen others. Two employees of the Brentwood mail facility died in the attacks. The Bureau of Prison offices and many of the other DC offices received their mail from the Brentwood facility.

The Beltway sniper attacks began one year later, on October 2, when the DC metropolitan area and the I-95 corridor south, became the target of two snipers. Ten people were killed and three critically injured in those attacks in various locations. Two of the victims were shot and one killed in Fredericksburg. The area was once again on alert. High school football games were canceled, and other events were impacted by the sniper attacks.

One of the saddest things about the move from Colorado to Virginia was not being able to take our dogs with us. Snickers had developed an illness and needed constant attention. We found her a home with a loving family who could give her the love and care that she needed. Wolfgang stayed with her.

We would not be without a dog for long however. Soon after we settled in our new home, Lola joined our family. Lola was a spirited Chihuahua pup. A few months later, while on a trip to the veterinary office with Lola, Karen and the girls met another Chihuahua. The vet was trying to find a new family for this dog but was not having success, and his future was much in doubt. His life had not been easy. He apparently had been mistreated and abused by previous owners. He was very timid, withdrawn, and uncomfortable around people.

They brought him home and named him Blue because of the tint of his coat. He bonded with Lola very quickly, though she was not thrilled to have competition for affection. Lola and Blue would have three litters of puppies together. The last pup of the last litter was the most unusual of all the pups, and somehow, Jenny and Kelly managed to keep this one. He was a long-haired Chihuahua pup with a white coat and black markings around his eyes, back, and feet. He was unanimously given the name Bandit.

Each of the dogs had very distinctive personalities with Lola, the unquestioned queen of the house. Blue, our rescue dog, was coming out of his shell and displaying amazing loyalty and contentment. And though we did not know it at the time, Bandit's mission would become, in part, that of a therapy dog.

APPLE, APPLE

There was a knock at the front door early one Saturday morning in May, a few years ago. One of the two sheriff's deputies standing on the porch asked Karen, who had responded to the knock and opened the door, if her husband was home. She nervously responded that he was, and they told her that they needed to talk to both of us. We invited them into the house with a gracious but worried apprehension.

As most parents instinctively know, it is usually not good news when law enforcement officers come to your home, especially that early in the morning. They asked if we knew where our two daughters were. "Jennifer is here," I responded while pointing to a lump of blankets on the living room floor where Jennifer, on a sleeping bag and wrapped in blankets, was fast asleep. A friend of hers was asleep on the couch. After checking Kelly's bedroom and then looking in the driveway to see that the car she was driving was not there, I told them that Kelly was not yet home.

"Are you sure that's your daughter?" he asked. I walked over to where Jennifer was fast asleep, buried deep in the blankets, and I lifted the blanket up so that I could see a face, and to my great relief, I confirmed that, yes, that is indeed Jennifer.

We told them that we thought Kelly was at a friend's house, but we would have to confirm that before saying for sure. It was not unusual for Kelly to spend the night at a friend's house. She would almost always call, or Karen would call her, and let us know what her plans were and when she would be home. She had talked with Karen on the phone earlier that morning, and we believed that she was still at the friend's house.

Kelly had moved back home four months earlier after attending Liberty University in Lynchburg, Virginia, for three semesters. She had enjoyed her time at Liberty and had earned good grades but had been sick quite a bit after Christmas and had come home to fully recover. She planned to return to Liberty or transfer to a different school for the fall semester.

"You and your wife need to sit down," he said. "We have something to tell you. Kelly has been injured in a horrific car accident and has been airlifted by helicopter to a level one trauma center. She is still alive, at last report, but has some serious injuries." The deputy had been told that the outlook for her surviving the crash was bleak at best, and we should leave to go to the hospital as soon as possible. We silently stared at the officer with a disbelieving look on our faces while trying to absorb the shock of what he was telling us.

He had asked about both of our daughters because the driver's license of Jenny had been found in the floor of the crushed car. They thought that Jenny might have been in the passenger seat during the accident and that she may have been thrown from the car or become disoriented, as a result of the accident, and walked away into the darkness. They had conducted an unsuccessful search of the area for Jenny.

We asked the officers a few questions about her condition, and they told us what they knew. She had sustained head injuries, internal injuries, and injuries to both feet. We tried to wake Jennifer so that she could go to the hospital with us, but when she appeared too sleepy and groggy, it was best to let her sleep. We told her that Kelly had been in a car accident and that we were going to the hospital. She softly acknowledged, and we hurriedly left the house and began a forty-five-minute drive to the hospital in Northern Virginia.

The drive seemed to take forever, and all other troubles disappeared as I focused on the thoughts and fears racing through our minds about the condition of our oldest daughter. We prayed together and silently, asking God to spare her life. A terror gripped my body as I briefly thought about the possibility that we might face a decision about donating our child's organs to save other lives. *No*, I thought. *Don't think about that. She will be okay.*

When we finally arrived and made our way to the trauma unit, we were taken to a waiting area where one of the surgeons would speak with us. He described her injuries to us, told us that she was in an induced coma, answered our questions, and told us what to expect when we went to her bedside. If she survived, she would need surgery on both of her feet and ankles, which had been crushed.

The emotion of the moment was overwhelming as we arrived at her bedside to see her pale, motionless body wrapped tightly in warm blankets. Medical equipment surrounded her, and tubes protruded from her mouth and nose. It was a horrible sight for anyone to encounter, but this was our little girl, and we felt helpless and unable to give her comfort. We did not know if she could hear us, but we talked to her and prayed for her as she lay comatose.

As we looked at her medical chart, we noticed that the name they had given Kelly was Apple, Apple. Kelly had been admitted to the hospital under the name Apple, Apple because the staff on the Flight for Life helicopter who transported her to the trauma center did not know her identity. As we would soon discover, all of her initial paperwork and hospital records would identify her as Apple, Apple.

After an hour or so at her bedside, I left the trauma unit and walked down the hallway to a nearby waiting room hoping to find a place to pray and try to process the events that had so quickly unfolded. I needed to consider the many new tasks that suddenly needed our attention. I was quite relieved to see that there were no other people in the waiting room.

After just a few minutes, a phone sitting on a nearby table began to ring. Although no one knew I was there and there was still no one else in the room, I picked up the phone to see if I could assist the caller. The voice on the other end was Jennifer's friend who had been at the house when we left. Jennifer had woken up and realized that we had told her that we were going to the hospital. She could not remember which hospital, and she and her friend began frantically to make calls to the many area hospitals to see if they could locate us.

No hospital that Jenny called had a record of Kelly being admitted. Even the one we were in had no record of Kelly since she had been admitted under the name Apple, Apple. The operator at this hospital had for some reason decided to transfer the call to this waiting room, where I just happened to be, and just happened to answer the phone.

This must have been another "God moment." What are the odds of me being in that waiting room and answering the phone at the exact moment that Jennifer called? But it happened. I told Jennifer where we were, and she, along with two friends, rushed to be at her sister's side.

Later that evening, as Karen and I reentered the hospital, we passed by the chapel and almost instinctively went inside, to the front, where we knelt down and began to pray for our daughter. Tears began to run down my face for the first time since we learned of the news.

I recalled the story my mom had told about praying in the Vanderbilt chapel when I was in surgery after swallowing a bead when I was twenty-one months old. The bead aspirated into my right lung and required surgery to remove the lower lobe. After much prayer, she began to sing a hymn. "God of grace and God of glory…grant us wisdom, grant us courage for the facing of this hour, for the facing of this hour." It was a story, and a song, that I would remember often over the years, particularly during difficult times.

I certainly needed wisdom and courage for this moment. Why did this happen was the thought that kept racing my mind? God is so good. What did I do wrong that put my child in harm's way? Why can't I make this go away?

I realized my mom must have asked the same questions when I was in surgery so long ago. I didn't think my heart could break more than it was breaking, yet it did. It wasn't until I was a grown man, a father of two girls, that I fully realized the guilt that my mom must have carried all those many years: guilt that she need not have carried.

She was not to blame for the allergic reaction to sulfa drugs that damaged my kidneys or the bead I swallowed that damaged my lung. Surely she knew that. To me it was just the way it happened—nobody's fault. I never conceived an idea of blaming anyone, especially my mom, for anything that happened.

It was too late to tell her that she should have had no regrets. I would love to have the chance to tell her that I forgive her if that is what she needed to hear. But she had died a few years earlier, preceded by my father. Karen and I were alone in the chapel asking God for courage to face this hour.

Though it was a progressive series of lessons, not fully realized until adulthood, I have learned firsthand that forgiveness plays a significant role in the physical and spiritual healing of the human body.

All families have their tragedies and illnesses, which they must bear. Ours is no different. My brothers and sister and their families have each endured sickness, accidents, surgeries, pain, and suffering within their own family.

Now I was called to be there for our child just as my parents had been there for me. The recovery for Kelly was a tough road. She had sustained a traumatic brain injury, injuries to internal organs, and many cuts and bruises. The most serious injuries were to her feet with bones in both feet and ankles being crushed, resulting in permanent injury.

Kelly's condition improved from critical to stable fairly quickly, and thankfully, there was never a point where we were given counsel or guidance about the process of the donation of her organs. I still find it a difficult question to consider.

Kelly and Jennifer both were, and still are, registered organ donors. *What if she had not survived and her wish to be an organ donor became reality?* As is the case with so many families who face this type of tragedy, in the terrible circumstances of death, several other people may receive the gift of life.

FOREVER GRATEFUL

The surgeon showed us the X-rays as he described the extensive injuries to Kelly's ankles. He told us that they would perform at least two separate surgeries, one on each ankle, on different days, to try to restore the bone structure and save her feet from amputation. Numerous pins, bolts, and screws were surgically implanted in both feet in an attempt to allow her to keep her feet and to restore some mobility.

Kelly was released from the hospital after seventeen days. She would slowly recover from most of her injuries, but many of the bones in her feet and ankles had been crushed. She would not be able to put weight on either foot for at least six weeks, and then she would walk with the aid of crutches for a few weeks. Her family was there to help her through this time.

Modifications were needed within our home to accommodate these new circumstances. Our home had three levels with three sets of stairs, and Kelly's room was on the lower level. We acquired a hospital bed and put it in the living room where she could be nearest to assistance as needed.

She learned to scoot around the house and up a staircase to get to the kitchen and bathroom. A wheelchair, crutches, and other medical equipment was rented or purchased. These types of mobility limitations would be difficult for anyone, and they were particularly difficult for a young, single woman. Her life would not be the same again.

She endured months of physical and pain management therapy, but perhaps the best and most effective therapy during the most difficult days came from her best friend, Bandit. Still a young pup himself, with no worries in the world, his eternal enthusiasm and unfaltering love inspired Kelly like nothing else short of her faith could possibly have done. He stayed with her and cuddled with her and loved her when she was in the worst of pain. And he did not care or love her any less because her feet were broken.

Pets seem to help people with chronic illness. Bandit reminded me of Butch, a red- or rust-colored Doberman pinscher pup given to me by my parents about the time I started dialysis. I called him Butch because he reminded me of a boxer we had as children. His muscular body and stunning appearance turned every head. Friend and foe alike paused upon approach, certain they wanted no fight with this giant.

While I was on kidney dialysis and after the transplant, when I was slowly regaining strength and health, he was there to challenge me to run faster, jump higher, get stronger, and never take life for granted. He was the definition of health, and his strength, vitality, boundless energy, enthusiasm, and love of life could bring a tear to the eye of young and old alike. But this was a gentle giant, and he seemed to think that I was pretty cool too.

After a long summer, Kelly began to walk again, with a conspicuous limp, but the initial surgeries on her feet were not the final solution to her pain and mobility concerns. Arthritis developed and reached its end stage quickly in her right foot to the point where the pain was excruciating at times. She would still need the aid of a wheelchair or crutches during the most difficult days.

Kelly sought the opinions of several foot and ankle specialists throughout the region. Most recommended either ankle fusion surgery or amputation as the only possibilities to improve mobility and quality of life. If the ankle was fused, she might not experience all or most of the pain from arthritis but would no longer be able to move the foot up and down. And the surgery is not always successful in relieving the pain.

Both options would permanently restrict her mobility and prevent all hope of returning to the active lifestyle she enjoyed before the accident. Kelly chose to continue her fight for as long as possible without undergoing ankle fusion surgery or amputation of her foot.

A little more than five years after Kelly's accident, Jennifer was working at her job as a teller at a local bank when a customer began to describe a terrible auto accident that had recently occurred. All of a sudden, and seemingly from nowhere, emotion took Jennifer by storm and came pouring out as she flashed back to that day. She could not hold back the tears and could not describe to others the feelings about her sister that was so overwhelming to her. We are all still affected by the events of that day.

Eventually, the mobility issues, pain, and associated problems became unbearable, and she sought additional advice for treatment. An appointment was scheduled with Paul Cooper, MD, orthopedic surgeon and founder and director of the Foot and Ankle Center at MedStar Georgetown University Hospital. He performed surgery on Kelly's right foot, removing the pins and other hardware.

The surgery also included the use of allograft: a gift of donated heart tissue, bone, or connective tissue. Donated bone is stored in a tissue bank until needed. Allograft procedures would not be possible without the final act of generosity and kindness of donors and the support of their families. The decision to donate, whether made by the donor or his family, was done in the hope of helping others in need. Most families never learn the difference their gifts have made to recipients.

LifeNet Health Tissue Development is an organization that facilitates communication between anonymous donors and recipients, if desired. A recipient may write an anonymous letter of gratitude to the recipients and then send the letter to LifeNet. It will then be forwarded to the donor family who will then be made aware of the hope their loved ones gift has given to someone in need.

Kelly received bone from three separate donors for the surgery, Cancellous Cubes, and two separate Iliac Crest Wedges. After the surgery, LifeNet gave one card to Kelly for each of the three donors. Each card had an ID number, a code, and the allograft serial number that would identify the anonymous donor to LifeNet.

It is hoped that at some point in the future, Dr. Cooper can implant the third-generation Scandinavian Total Ankle Replacement (STAR) system device, a three-component implant approved by the Food and Drug Administration in 2009. Dr. Cooper became the first surgeon in the United States to implant the revolutionary STAR system device soon after its approval.

Our family will be forever grateful to the donors and their families for this precious gift. It has given Kelly the opportunity to avoid amputation of her foot, to continue the healing process, and to walk again without pain. It provides hope that in the future, she may receive a total ankle replacement, which could further restore her mobility.

INVICTUS

Our family has been through the transplant process as both an organ donor and an organ recipient. Yet this incident with Kelly taught me a very important lesson. The decision to donate organs and tissues is very personal and very important. One needs to know as much as possible about the donation process before the need to make a decision arises. This is the only way to make the right decision for yourself or a loved one.

The dramatic developments in science and medicine that have allowed for the gift of life for hundreds of thousands over the last fifty years, have, for some, created a new controversy about the definition of death.

Kelly described her feelings about the accident and her recovery in a paper she wrote for a college class she took many months after the accident. The paper was an analysis of the poem *Invictus* by William Ernest Henley with comments about how it applied to her life.

Kelly writes:

> Recently, I was introduced to a poem that truly inspired me and confirmed personal feelings I thought were rare. Although the word *use* and *imagery* in poems usually confuses me, I completely related to William Ernest Henley's *Invictus* with a stunning ease. I will discuss the poem and what it meant to me personally as it reminds me of one of the most difficult times of my life.

The narrator, in *Invictus*, is going through a dark time, with many threats and dangers lurking about. Contradictory to the fear intended by his enemies, he's found great supernatural strength and fearlessness. This reminded me of a time when I was in a bad car accident and all odds were against me ever walking again, but my faith was more tangible than I'd ever known it could be, and I felt an amazing sense of security that I would recover no matter what!

Even in the opening lines, "In the night that covers me, Black as the pit from pole to pole," I can picture the time in the hospital waiting eagerly to leave but knowing I was to be on bed rest, or in a wheel chair, for who knew how long. I couldn't see the future, not even the distant future, because the doctors didn't even know what to expect.

From every angle, there was no certainty. But the narrator proceeds to say, "I thank whatever gods may be for my unconquerable soul." At that same time in the hospital, I was so grateful to be alive and really felt like a survivor. And I recognized this strength as a blessing from God. I felt that he would carry me through this experience. For some reason, he just didn't let me worry about the future. It was a train of thought alien to me. I was so grateful for that assurance and that it kept me optimistic at the oddest of times.

The accident was the result of being at the wrong place at the wrong time, but I couldn't go back and change it for a redo. My situation wouldn't change. Everyone, it seemed, was

> curious as to what attitude I would have about the daunting new challenges that lay ahead. It sounds to me as if it would have been easy for the narrator to have been distraught in one form or another. Instead, he says:
>
> In the fell clutch of circumstance
> I have not winced nor cried aloud.
> Under the bludgeonings of chance
> My head is bloody, yet unbowed.

It's funny because my head was bloodied due to windshield glass. Even with the stitches on my forehead, it would often bleed, reminding me of the scars to come. I really admire the way Henley expressed bravery in the face of adversity.

In the hospital, the pain was bad, and I knew that dealing with the dramatic adjustments to my life would be just as hard. Then the doctors had to warn me how there will be less medicine to kill the pain when I leave. They emphasized that I wouldn't be going back to the way things used to be. Simple things, like walking downstairs to my room, were now impossible, and they couldn't guess the other simplicities I'd have to kiss good-bye.

The feelings I had in the hospital in relation to my release were like when he said, "Beyond this place of wrath and tears Looms but the Horror of the shade." It's like, the worst may only get worse, but who knows? Such possibility in itself can be quite debilitating. That's what God's enemy would have wanted me to think. But thanks to God, I could feel more like the way this man did in the poem. He says, "And yet the menace of the years finds and shall find me unafraid."

I remember when they told me that it would be a very long recovery and that I couldn't even try to take a step for at least six months. All the plans I had, all the responsibility I'd already incurred, were shaved to a bare minimal. Those times of recovery would be filled with pain and difficult days and nights. And I knew that I would have to work very hard and let the sweat take over if I wanted to recuperate and recover as much as possible. There were certain rules, exercises, stretches, and guidelines I had to follow, just like when the narrator said,

> It matters not how strait the gate,
> How charged with punishments the scroll,
> I am the master of my fate:
> I am the captain of my soul.

I knew that the future was in my hands. If I was dedicated to the healing process, then healing would come. And I knew that if I let fear take over and depression sink in, I would never come out of this dark and lonely time.

I'm so glad to hear that someone else has seen life this way. And that we are not victims of circumstances, but they are ours to own. That God blesses us, and he will carry us and give us strength to walk to our fate. *Invictus* is a beautiful poem of triumph over fear and grasping one's own course to take one where one may want to go.

THE CABIN

> A family is a wondrous thing; and we will rejoice in remembering our yearly get togethers in a "cabin" where we catch up on our year's events and plan for things to come. It is the tie that binds our hearts together to weather every storm.
>
> —Mildred Cooper Russell

The cabin was busy with children playing in one area while the adults, in stiff competition, were at different tables, playing some of the many games brought to this year's reunion. Two long tables of snacks, many especially prepared for this occasion, lined one wall of the kitchen. This night's supper was finished, the dishes washed, and the kitchen cleaned. The entire group would come together later in the evening for a gift exchange and then a round or two of charades.

Fast-forward to the twenty-first century and find the family gathered together all in one place deep in the mountains of Georgia or North Carolina. They have planned for time off work, saved the money, and traveled hundreds of miles, in some cases to spend as much time together as possible over the next five or six days. Three generations descended from Bill and June Cooper keep the tradition of gathering together alive and well.

The cabin was large enough to comfortably house all of the families represented. There were enough bedrooms and beds for everyone, a full bath for every bedroom, and separate heating and air conditioning for each room. From the porch, the shadows of the distant mountain peaks could be seen glimmering in the clear, cold lake in the valley below.

A bonfire, when the sun sets, will burn for hours with the wood collected in the surrounding forests. The young boys, with their new night vision goggles, will venture through the woods playing, with imaginations running wild. These have been precious times as we have watched our families grow and begin families of their own.

The first few reunions were held near Helen, Georgia, which is located in the mountains of Northern Georgia. The family was gathered together there on New Year's Eve as the whole world celebrated the arrival of the twenty-first century. Depending on the location, the New Year might be celebrated with fireworks of various sorts. It has become a tradition for all to gather together around the television, with a beverage of choice in hand, as the countdown begins to usher in each New Year.

Horseback riding and a round of golf, for those interested, are usually on one day's agenda. Snow skiing, billiards, and ping-pong have been included in the activities at some sites.

The location of the reunion has changed from time to time as the search for suitable accommodations is unending. The current location has seemed to fit the needs of everyone quite well for now and has been the destination for the last several years.

The biggest difference from the reunions back in the day, other than the fact that we are all under one roof and for several days, seems to be the multitude of cell phones, laptop computers, tablets, video games, and a multitude of other electronic gadgets of all types that have sprung up in recent years.

Communication with the outside world is readily available through social media and the Internet. It's a strange sight to see the youngest to the oldest, sitting around, deep in concentration, staring at the screen of a small device, and communicating with friends back home.

But there is only one television. That makes for a stiff challenge when there are many ballgames to watch. And there is allegiance now to many different teams confusing and challenging old boundaries. Ole Miss, Kentucky, and the St. Louis Cardinals are not the only teams in town anymore.

The four children of Bill and June, now lovingly called the originals, and their spouses have somehow now become the elder statesmen. Billy, now retired, earned his master's degree and taught mathematics at Meridian Community College in Meridian, Mississippi, for more than thirty years.

He has become the family historian and has maintained connections with relatives in Mississippi and other parts of the country, as much as possible, over the years. A family genealogy is traced to the earliest years of colonial American and to the families of Europe.

Gayle has been by his side the entire time as they raised their family. She was a working mom and a stellar employee at several jobs before retiring from the railroad. She, like our mom, has a great love of and talent with all types of flowers and landscaping.

Their daughters, Lara Gayle and Karen Kelly, are married to kind, loving, and hardworking husbands. They each work outside the home and are very active in their children's lives as they raise their beautiful families.

Lara Gayle and Jacob Edward have three children: Jordan Elaine, Luke Cooper, and Jacob Thomas. Karen Kelly and William Earl have two children: Jessica Kay and William Brant.

Mildred and Rusty have resided in Gainesville, Florida, for over thirty years. They have traveled to dozens of countries around the world and throughout the United States primarily in their capacity as evangelists and teachers. Mildred was a home school mom and has volunteered for years in her community.

They have a son, Jason Matthew, and a daughter, Rebekah Elizabeth. Becka recently graduated from the University of Florida. Jason has a daughter, Abigail Sephrenia.

Ed and Laurie have lived in Nashville since 1982. Together they have raised three children: Katheryn Meg, Caroline Grey, and William Clayton. Katie earned a master's degree from Vanderbilt University. Caroline earned a master's degree from the University of Kentucky and Clay attended Georgetown University Law School.

Katie is married to William Christie (Tie) Watkins IV, and Caroline is married to Sean Jamison Huddleston.

Luke and Caroline had surgery as infants, so they Ed and I have similar zipper scars.

Karen and I have two daughters: Kelly Elaine and Jennifer Joy. Kelly has attended Liberty University, and Jennifer is preparing for nursing school. It looks like we may finally have a nurse in the family. Jennifer was recently engaged to Anthony Eddy Cordero. Anthony attended his first cabin reunion during the most recent gathering and was welcomed, with open arms, into the family circle.

When Billy and Gayle moved to Meridian, we would go see them around Christmas time, or they would travel to Paducah to be with family. Even as the years have quickly passed and we have each moved quite a distance from one another, we have all made an effort to gather together as often as possible.

The tradition of our family reunion is traced as far back as any of us can remember. Almost every summer, our family would make the six-hour drive to our mother's hometown of Carthage, Mississippi, for a family reunion the first Sunday in June.

The grounds of the old family church were the setting. The lovingly maintained church building was opened for the special occasion, and the business of the families was conducted inside.

The newest family cemetery at Rocky Hill was only a few yards away. Here we would travel to bury loved ones. There are other cemeteries, some very old and difficult to find, in the area where relatives have been laid to rest. Plans were finalized at the reunions to build a fence around the cemetery at Rocky Hill and ensure that it is maintained in perpetuity.

Some years, there were new headstones, and those were usually viewed first. Some years, there were more than others. It was a history lesson though we did not realize that at the time. War heroes, pastors, businessmen, teachers, homemakers, doctors, politicians, and children who died too young occupy the grounds. Maybe even a lawyer or two. Many generations had settled this part of the country after migrating from the former colonies.

It was at the reunions where we learned firsthand how sweltering hot Mississippi summers could be. Though shaded by huge trees, there was no place to escape the stifling heat. Plenty of food and drinks were a nice distraction. The adults talked and the children played. The oldest were afforded the greatest honor, and the children must be respectful to everyone.

Billy, Gayle, and the girls continued to attend the family reunion in Carthage over the years and still do. They also attend the annual cousin's day in October. The rest of us have only been able to attend those reunions occasionally though the heart is always there.

After Billy and Gayle were married, they would celebrate Christmas at Mom and Dad's house with our immediate family. Later, partly due to circumstances, the family would travel to Meridian to celebrate after Christmas at Billy and Gayle's house. Later, as our families grew and spread out, gathering together for reunions was more difficult and was abandoned for a time.

Lara and Karen were the primary inspiration and driving force for restoring the tradition that continues today. On the wall of our bedroom hangs a precious gift received by Mildred, Ed, and I from Gayle and Billy. It is a picture of the four of us together with a descriptive quote underneath the picture. It reads:

> Our family is
> a circle of strength and
> love—With every birth and
> every union the circle grows.
> Every joy shared adds more love.
> Every crisis faced makes
> the circle stronger. (C. Blaine)

JOURNEY OF MIRACLES

Mildred was working at a small clothing manufacturing company, Normandy Frocks, when she and Henry Russell began dating shortly after the family moved to the Stanley Road home. Rusty had noticed Mildred at the church where his father was the pastor and asked Tom if she was dating anyone. With encouragement from Tom and some friends, they began dating. Shortly afterward, Bob and Rose Weiner moved to Paducah to follow up with the young people who had been saved at the revival meetings at Broadway Methodist Church.

After a few months, Bob and Rose sought a permanent place where they could hold Bible studies and praise meetings. With help from some adults in the community who believed in their vision and ministry, the Maranatha Christian Center held its first services on Monday October 9, 1972. (Rose Russell Weiner is Rusty's sister.) The center was established as a nondenominational youth center for the young people of the area. Bob was only twenty-six years old at the time, and Rose was twenty-four. They were both new Christians, having been saved for little more than two years.

From its humble beginnings, the ministry of the Maranatha Center grew and expanded. It would soon become one of the first and largest organizations of its kind on college campuses in the United States. It would soon become a one-of-a-kind ministry with influence that would reach throughout the United States and around the world.

The first summer the center was open, 1973, thirty high school and college young people were added to the staff, dedicating their summer to ministry. One team held weekly Bible classes in the various housing projects and apartment complexes in the area. The classes were held outdoors for children from ages seven to thirteen. They featured Bible stories, songs, games, and refreshments.

Other teams featured street evangelism, newsletter and newspaper ministry, follow-up ministry, and music ministry. They sang and spoke at church camps, Boy Scout camps, summer festivals, shopping centers, and other venues.

Maranatha became a certified drug prevention center and established a twenty-four-hour hotline funded by the Mayor's Committee on Drug Prevention and thought to be the first of its kind in the region.

Part of the initial mission of the ministry was to address and help combat the growing drug and alcohol issues in area schools. Ministry and certified hotline counselors would frequently receive requests for assistance from parents and students concerning these and other issues. Some hotline calls might result from someone contemplating suicide or from overwhelming feelings of loneliness, hopelessness, or despair. Incidents of domestic violence and threats of other types of destructive behaviors were also common reasons for a call to the hotline.

One day, in 1974, Mom collapsed at home and was rushed to the hospital. She was bleeding internally, but the doctor did not know why. She needed many pints of blood to replace the blood she was losing every day. The prayer hotline at church was contacted for prayer. Dozens of people from the Maranatha church gave blood in an overwhelming demonstration of love and compassion. Hospital staff was astonished at the tremendous number of volunteer donors. Then one day, the bleeding increased, and she was rushed to surgery. The doctor did not believe she would survive; he did not know what the source of bleeding was. After prayer for her, the doctor, a Christian man, discovered the source, a perforated ulcer. He was able to perform surgery and save her life.

As Mom was rushed to surgery, Rusty went to the hospital chapel to pray for his mother-in-law. The Lord gave him the Scripture Ezekiel 16:6, "And when I passed by you and saw you squirming in your own blood, I said to you in your blood, 'Live!'" Rusty declared in prayer that Mom would live and then shared it with the family. We knew then that she would indeed live.

(Though the context of this verse applies to Israel, when spoken by God in answer to prayer, it became the Living Word for our situation.)

Mom did survive that incident, and once again, the prayer of faith, along with her indomitable spirit, was thought to have turned the tide in her favor. The young people of this ministry would become known for their belief in the miraculous healing power of God.

Mildred began working in the church office shortly after the ministry began. After much prayer, Rusty made a decision to enter full-time ministry. He left Paducah to attend Christ for the Nations Bible College in Dallas, Texas. A year later, after completing his studies, he returned to Paducah with a strong passion for ministry.

The couple was married in 1974 at the church to which the ministry had recently moved. Rusty's father performed the ceremony. They have served together in the ministry ever since.

In the early eighties, they began a newsletter entitled *Journey of Miracles*, which described the remarkable events occurring as a result of their ministry. The newsletter has gone the way of most paper news and is now sent via e-mail. It is a wonderful way of keeping in touch with disciples and supporters. Especially important is the prayer team, a vital part of the success of the ministry.

Rusty and Mildred left Paducah in 1976 to help start an outreach to the University of Georgia in Athens. They remained as senior pastors for two and a half years. It was a special time in their lives. The church was truly a family, a very close-knit group of believers seeking to know Jesus more deeply. Rusty and Mildred are still friends with many of the people from that time in their lives.

Their next adventure in ministry took them to Oxford, England. They participated in a two-month outreach at Oxford University in July and August of 1979. Mildred and Rusty were leaders of the team that remained in Oxford and established a campus ministry at that historic university. Though unique, that ministry was also a special time of ministry, friendships, and building of faith.

The couple returned to the states in the early eighties and, from their home in Florida, traveled together as a team, often with their children, to minister in churches throughout the United States.

In the mideighties, they returned to England and Ireland with the children for a two-and-a-half week tour. Rusty spoke at a couple of lunchtime meetings sponsored by The Bible Society the fellowship club on the University College–Dublin campus. The couple's ministry continued day and night with Rusty eventually losing his voice for a while. Mildred filled in undeterred. She preached for two days on God's purpose for his church and our responsibility for self-government and diligence in being obedient to God. Her messages were so well received that everyone wanted a copy of her teaching.

Mildred said she enjoyed the opportunity that God provided for her to minister in Dublin. She then offered a word of encouragement to women everywhere to be prepared when God provides the opportunity. The family then traveled to Peacehaven, England, where pastors, John and Heather Cairns served as hosts at their ministry, Abundant Life.

Maranatha Ministries would move its headquarters to Gainesville, Florida, in 1981, and the church in Paducah would close a short time after that. Maranatha Christian Churches Inc. was officially dissolved in 1990 after eighteen years of ministry on college campuses and communities throughout the United States and around the world.

The corporate structure of the ministry that had developed over the years became too restrictive to the large number of churches that had been planted. In a November 1989 staff meeting, Bob Weiner proposed that the corporation be dissolved, the international office in Gainesville closed, and that the local churches and ministries receive complete autonomy. The Maranatha churches, however, either closed, continued independently, or merged with other church networks.

The historic fall of the Berlin Wall that separated communist East Germany from West Germany had occurred just a few months earlier. Bob Weiner believed that his calling was now to Russia and the Eastern block countries. Rusty and Mildred and Bob and Rose traveled to Russia and other Eastern European countries extensively over the next several years.

The Weiners founded Christian Youth International and conducted several conferences in Russia that trained thousands of Christian leaders for ministry in Russia and other former communist countries. Students from all over the communist world and from many different types of churches attended the conferences. Many were international students studying in Russia from the other fourteen former republics of the Soviet Union. And there were students from Africa and Asia as well as Eastern Europe. Rusty participated in the conferences, teaching a workshop on the gifts of the Spirit. Many miracles resulted through the lives of those who attended. It was a time of great harvest in the open and hungry harvest field of Russia.

After the dissolution of Maranatha Christian Ministries, Rusty and Mildred sought the Lord for direction for the next phase of their ministry. They formed Miracle Life Ministries based in Gainesville, Florida. The ministry is an evangelistic prophetic missionary organization helping to establish new churches and supporting existing churches in prophetic evangelism.

The Lord opened the door to Singapore in 2002. Rusty's Asia division is called Miracle Life Ministries Asia. Three main focuses for Miracle Life Ministries are the three *m*'s: miracles, mentoring, and missions. Rusty's main ministry now is to Asia including the countries of Singapore, Indonesia, Malaysia, Nepal, Hong Kong, and China.

Rusty has traveled to fifty-seven countries preaching the Gospel, praying for the sick, and ministering in churches, home groups, Bibles studies, and hospitals. He has a heart for God and for his people. He is a willing and obedient servant, always on call to those who need his ministry. Mildred has responsibilities at home, but she travels with him some and prays for him always. Mildred recently preached at Saint Andrew's Cathedral in Singapore.

NO GREATER LOVE

Choosing to become an organ donor reflects one's deepest beliefs about the sanctity and importance of life. Some find it an easy decision; others want to be assured they're doing the right thing by their faith. And so they look to others for counsel. Though the answers vary from one religion and denomination to another, research has found that the vast majority of religions do support donation and transplantation. Sometimes the decision to donate organs has to be made at the most tragic and confusing moments a family will encounter.

Many people of faith believe that since God created the human body, it is God who heals. It is also recognized that modern science and medicine play a significant role in the health and well-being of an individual. A 1992 resolution from one denomination stated, "Donation is to be encouraged, assuming appropriate safeguards against hastening death and determination of death by reliable criteria."

For tens of thousands of transplant recipients, the dramatic improvement in the quality and length of life is undeniable. Organ and tissue transplantation has transformed many lives around the world. Thousands of donors, donor families, and recipients and families have attended and successfully competed in transplant Olympic Games over the last twenty years.

Though the first successful kidney transplant was performed in the 1950s, it is almost impossible to find complete records on a combined national basis before 1984 when a national organ allocation system was implemented by an act of congress. We do know that a few transplant recipients have survived more than forty years, and the numbers exceeding thirty years is growing quickly.

The Quarter Century Club is an organization started several years ago by George Franklin, a kidney transplant recipient. The club has several dozen members, all of whom have survived twenty-five years or more after transplant. Quite a few have exceeded thirty years, and at least a couple of them are forty years posttransplant. The club has an Internet group site and a Facebook page where the members correspond with one another about the many topics of interest relevant to such an elite group.

They have, as a group, attended several of the national Transplant Games over the years and gathered for a dinner cruise where networking with peers and sharing stories of their life's journeys have helped create significant and lasting bonds of friendship.

They are also an important educational resource to researchers and professionals regarding current issues of transplantation. This unique club should continue to grow and prosper as, each year, more transplant recipients achieve the quarter century anniversary of their transplant.

Many of the members received their transplants before records of transplant donors and recipients were kept on a consolidated national basis. Records have been lost, and it is difficult to determine accurate statistics of transplants and surviving donors and recipients prior to 1984. An organization in California does maintain a fairly complete data base of pre-1984 transplants, but it is not a complete list.

The Quarter Century Club members provide an excellent sample for older transplant statistics. Advances in transplantation and medications including dosages and the varying side effects of each medication are common topics. Some individuals have encountered numerous and serious complications from long-term immunosuppression, such as loss of bone density or varying types of skin cancers. Others have encountered less serious issues.

Taking Flight: Inspirational Stories of Lung Transplantation—More Journeys is a wonderful book by Joanne Schum. The second edition of *Taking Flight*, together with the first book, contains hundreds of stories authored by lung recipients from around the world.

Organ transplantation in the United States is built on altruism and public trust. The organ allocation system in the United States is managed by the United Network for Organ Sharing (UNOS). The website organtransplants.org/understanding/unos/ describes the creation of UNOS.

In 1984, the National Organ Transplant Act established the Organ Procurement and Transplant Network (OPTN), a national organ sharing system to guarantee, among other things, fairness in the allocation of organs for transplant. Since 1984, the nonprofit United Network for Organ Sharing (UNOS) located in Richmond, Virginia, has operated the OPTN, under a contract with the Division of Transplantation in the Department of Health and Human Services.

UNOS maintains a central computer network containing the names of all patients waiting for kidney, heart, liver, lung, intestine, pancreas, and multiple-organ transplants; the UNOS Organ Center is staffed twenty-four hours a day to respond to requests to list patients, change status of patients, and help coordinate the placement of organs.

Living donors may donate a kidney, a lobe of the liver or lung, blood, marrow, peripheral blood stem cells, and umbilical cord blood. Deceased donors can donate multiple organs such as heart, kidneys, pancreas, lungs, liver, and small intestine. Tissues that may be donated include corneas, bone, heart valves, connective tissue, skin, and other tissues. The donation may be restricted to certain organs or tissues if that is their wish.

According to recent UNOS statistics:

- There were 116,511 waiting list candidates on November 9, 2012
- 18,986 transplants were performed November through August of 2012
- There were 9,502 donors November through August of 2012

The National Donor Memorial is located on the grounds of UNOS in Richmond, Virginia. Within the grounds of the garden are a Wall of Tears and a Wall of Names. There are dozens of donor family remembrance quilts throughout the country. Donor families are invited to create a square to honor their loved ones.

I was standing in the conference room of the secretary of the Department of Homeland Security at a reception and awards presentation ceremony when my thoughts began to wander. For the last six months, I had worked with staff at each of the twenty-three agencies within the department to train volunteers, speak at agency events, and encourage employees to donate money to the local, national, or international charity of their choice.

I had been appointed by the attorney general and the director of my agency to serve as a loaned executive to the organization that would run the federal government's annual fundraising efforts in the national capital area. Because the Department of Homeland Security had only recently been established, the task was particularly daunting.

The campaign ended successfully, exceeding goals, with a total of more than $55 million donated by employees from all of the agencies. It was quite a privilege to be a part of that team and to receive special recognition from the secretary. And as the reception progressed, I thought back over the years to transplant day and the gift of life from my brother that made my part in this day possible.

I have had the privilege of speaking at churches, several government agencies, and other organizations including to staff at the headquarters of the United Network for Organ Sharing (UNOS) about organ donation, donors, and recipients. My wife and I, like thousands of visitors, visited the National Donor Memorial and took time to remember the many donors and their sacrifice. I try to pass on the love that was shown to me, the gift of life, and the role that faith and friends play in that process.

REFUSE TO BE FEEBLE

> Let us hold fast the confession of our hope without wavering, for He who promised is faithful. And let us consider one another in order to stir up love and good works.
>
> —Hebrews 10:23–24

My family and I were privileged to meet Will Smith, owner and personal trainer at Will Smith's Better U Fitness Center at the first ever Virginia Transplant Games. Will is a champion bodybuilder and a kidney transplant recipient who chooses to be fit and offers inspiration and empathy to the people who turn to him with hope. His diet and weight training helped save his life not once but several times during a harrowing journey through a series of chronic illnesses. His clients call it will power or the power of will—an embodied joy that enables others to make the lifestyle changes necessary to reclaim their lives.

His clients include a woman who is legally blind and almost deaf, a man who had two heart attacks, a mother of five who dropped from a size 20 to a size 4, people dealing with depression, and others with challenges to overcome on their way to better health. In fact, it was one of Will's clients, Ellen Souviney, who donated a kidney out of gratitude for the new life she'd found in physical fitness. (From the synopsis of the upcoming book *The Power of Will* by Will Smith)

Trey, a former firefighter, forced by kidney disease to retire from his dream job with the city of Fredericksburg, is a friend still wrestling with the horrible effects of chronic kidney disease. He was fortunate to receive a second kidney transplant after the first one failed after a few years. The second transplanted kidney is also failing, and he is back on dialysis while waiting for a third gift of life.

Trey and I first met at the YMCA a few years ago when I overheard him discussing with some buddies his return to dialysis after his first transplant failed. I introduced myself, and we talked briefly and have kept in contact through social media.

He has married and enjoyed the birth of his first son. Broken bones from a brittle bone disease and a long assortment of additional devastating medical issues have kept him in and out of the hospital on a regular basis. He, like many dialysis patients, has watched helplessly as too many fellow dialysis friends have tragically died while waiting for a transplant.

He is a man of immense faith in God and attends church on a regular basis while also working a part-time job to help with family expenses. His story is not unique to human existence, and it could be one of terrible depression, heartbreak, and a life of misery. Yet he chose to live a life of positive inspiration, sharing the joy of abundant life through following Christ.

He recently mentioned his battle with depression while discussing the song "Perfect Peace by" Laura Story. "I think about the times of depression while on dialysis, and I think about the time when I was twenty-two years old just praying for the Lord to bring me home, tired of fighting daily on dialysis. This song wasn't around at the time, but the meaning was found for me in the Bible. While at my lowest, I found perfect peace in Jesus."

> And He said to me, "My grace is sufficient for you, for My strength is made perfect in weakness." Therefore most gladly I will rather boast in my infirmities, that the power of Christ may rest upon me. (2 Corinthians 12:9)

Attitude and faith in God can be one or our greatest weapons against the fear, depression, loneliness, and pain of a serious illness. I know that, when we ask, God can and does heal the physical and emotional problems we encounter during our earthly journey. It is one of several promises he gave us in the Holy Bible. Many books have been written and countless testimonies shared throughout the ages describing the innumerable ways that God has provided for individuals, including times of financial hardship and health challenges. Yet not everyone is healed.

The advances in medicine over just the last fifty years have been nothing less than a miracle as mankind discovers, through science and intellect, the seemingly endless possibilities of God's creation. Yet science, intellect, and medicine cannot cure every illness. Even the most advanced treatments using the most sophisticated technologies are often ineffective for a variable percentage of patients.

And even if we are cured of our current illness, through prayer and medicine, new challenges will certainly arise eventually with each new illness or accident. So what is our attitude to be? How do we endeavor to live life to its fullest and achieve the best health possible in our circumstance?

Science and faith have always been inseparable brothers throughout our human existence. As man understands more about God's spectacular creation, and begins to apply it in science and medicine, the human condition is improved. Yet, the unexplainable is, and has always been, part of our experience. The healing power of faith is a promise that is as valid today as it has ever been.

Russell Kelso Carter experienced serious heart problems long before medicine had advanced far enough to save his life. Yet, his physical heart condition, and his spiritual heart, was healed and he lived for several more decades. He would write several songs that would inspire generations to know and experience the healing power that comes from an understanding of God and His promises.

The promises of God are for everyone without exception. Sometimes we don't rely on them until there is great need and all else has failed.

Connie Ruth Christensen has written an article about the life of this man who wrote the great inspirational hymn "Standing on the Promises."

> Russell Kelso Carter (1849–1928) was a star athlete of a military academy and an excellent student academically, who went on to be

a successful teacher and coach. He then spent several years as an ordained Methodist minister, after which he went to medical school. He spent the last of his professional years as a doctor of medicine. Carter was also a musician and songwriter. In 1886, he co-edited Songs of Perfect Love with John Sweney (1837–1899), who wrote the music for such beloved songs as Beulah Land and Fill Me Now. This hymnbook included Carter's most famous hymn, Standing on the Promises.

Although Carter was a professed Christian most of his life, it wasn't until a crisis with his natural heart that he began to understand the reality and power of Bible promises. At age 30, his health was in critical condition and the physicians could do no more for him. Carter turned to God for help and healing.

He knelt and made a promise that healing or no, his life was finally and forever, fully consecrated to the service of the Lord. It was from that moment that the written Word of God became alive to Carter. He began to stand upon the promises of healing, determining to believe no matter what his physical condition, no matter how he felt. Over the course of the next several months his strength returned, and his heart was completely healed! Carter lived another healthy 49 years.

The hymn Carter had written several years before his healing miracle became more than words and music to him. Standing on the Promises became an integral part of his life.

This hymn continues to inspire and to also motivate me, especially in the many troubled times. Billy, Mildred, Ed and I, and our families have been tremendously blessed, throughout the years, and there is much for which to be thankful. It has not been a journey without many trials and tribulations along the way. There will be many more challenges to meet and overcome in the future. With trust in God, knowing that tomorrow is promised to no one, we will continue to trust in the promises of God.

STANDING ON THE PROMISES

Hymn by Russell Kelso Carter
Published 1886, public domain

Standing on the promises of Christ my King,
Through eternal ages let His praises ring,
Glory in the highest, I will shout and sing,
Standing on the promises of God.
Refrain:
Standing, standing,
Standing on the promises of God my Savior;
Standing, standing,
I'm standing on the promises of God.
Standing on the promises that cannot fail,
When the howling storms of doubt and fear assail,
By the living Word of God I shall prevail,
Standing on the promises of God.
Refrain
Standing on the promises I now can see
Perfect, present cleansing in the blood for me;

Standing in the liberty where Christ makes free,
Standing on the promises of God.
Refrain
Standing on the promises of Christ the Lord,
Bound to Him eternally by love's strong cord,
Overcoming daily with the Spirits sword,
Standing on the promises of God.
Refrain
Standing on the promises I cannot fall,
Listening every moment to the Spirit's call
Resting in my Savior as my all in all,
Standing on the promises of God.
Refrain

THE LEGACY OF LIFE

Mildred contributed the following for the conclusion to our story.

This is a small part of the story of the William Burt Cooper and June Elaine Waggoner Cooper family. It is both sad and sweet to us, deeply woven into the fabric that makes us, their children, who we are today. We have always been close, but Tom's illnesses, the transplant, the recovery and living of a full life have brought us together in a way that perhaps nothing else could have. We accept the miracle that God did in healing one brother through another one and are always thankful for his blessing on Tom and Ed and his protection of them as they continue to be productive adults, husbands, fathers, and brothers.

We began a tradition about ten years ago of getting together for a few days after Christmas. We do not live close to each other, except for Ed and Billy and Billy's youngest daughter for a few years, and we want to maintain our relationships. It took awhile to find a place big enough to accommodate us and our extended families, to be close enough to be accessible to all, and clean enough to satisfy the women.

We refer to this gathering as the cabin. We stay through the New Year in order to celebrate together another year of God's blessings, another year of great expectations, and thankfulness that we enjoy each other's company.

These gatherings include the consumption of much food, including about fifteen pounds of fudge, bourbon balls, homemade dips, cookies of all varieties, and other things we indulge in at the cabin. We play board games, card games, games with clues, and Dirty Santa. We sometimes work a jigsaw puzzle. We consume many cups of coffee and glasses of tea and soda. We talk, we laugh, and sometimes we cry, always desiring to encourage and inspire each other, believing that nothing can quench the love that we have managed to maintain over the years. It is our hope that our children will want to continue this tradition with their cousins after we originals are gone.

For the most part, there is little contention at the cabin. We have had our moments though, when feelings needed to be shared, when misunderstandings had to be talked through, when we needed to have a timeout in order to cool down and think through whatever was bothering us. Sometimes it takes a lot of work to overlook irritations and things we perceive as faults in others. I am happy to say that forgiveness is generous and usually readily given, that nothing has broken the bond that we have, the love we share, the desire to remain a strong and loving family. In this age that we live in, many families are broken and dysfunctional. We are not perfect, but we have a tradition of love and unity that we are thankful for, and we pray that we have modeled it well enough for our children to want carry it on.

We are wealthy indeed—rich in healing, rich in love, rich in God's grace, rich in his mercy, his kindness. Who could ask for more?

I wrote the following poem three or four years ago at the cabin. It is a small expression of who we are as a family.

A FAMILY IS A WONDROUS THING

By Mildred Cooper Russell

A family is a wondrous thing,
And we will rejoice in remembering
Our yearly get-togethers in a cabin
Where we catch up on our year's events
And plan for things to come.
It is the tie that binds our hearts together
To weather every storm.
A family is a wondrous thing,
Filled with laughter and
With love's sweet song
Sung in the small things
We do and in the things we share.
A family is memories, good and bad,
Happy and sad,
Which make us one no matter what comes our way.
A family is a wondrous thing,
Where love conquers everything
That would tear apart the ties that bind,
Where strength lies in forgiving
Our glaring faults and the subtle ones,
Where we encourage and inspire
Each other to move forward and reach upward
To achieve our dreams and goals.
Love conquers all and keeps us strong.

A family is a wondrous thing;
It is us.
May our lives live on in the younger ones,
And may our ties stay strong
So that many years from now
The Family Cooper will still be strong,
Still filled with love and laughter.
We will then live and laugh forever.

APPENDIX—TRANSPLANT STORIES

It is not always a simple decision to have your name added to a list for organ transplant. An organ transplant is not a cure for a disease. It is a treatment. Usually, it is the last treatment available to treat a disease.

There are many issues that can prevent one from qualifying for transplant. There is no guarantee that it will be successful or that the quality of life will be better afterward. The candidate knows the percentages of success and failure. They know the potential side effects of surgery and transplant medications. For various reasons, some may choose to decline a possible transplant.

STEVE'S STORY

My brother-in-law, Steve, recently received a pancreas and kidney transplant. Steve is the husband of Jeannie, my wife Karen's sister. Though Jeannie and Steve were both born and raised in Paducah, Steve has lived in Pullman, Washington, for more than thirty years. Karen's only other sibling and oldest sister, Elaine, and her husband, Mel, have also lived in Pullman where they have worked and raised their children.

After months of dialysis prior to the transplant, Steve has returned to health and has no more daily insulin shots. Steve continued working full-time while his life transitioned to dialysis and then to the waiting list.

Steve received the call four separate times to come to the hospital to prepare for transplant. Each time he and his wife, Jeannie, grabbed the go bag and made the four-hour car ride to Seattle. There are many concerns that must be addressed before the doctors on the transplant team will make the final decision to proceed with the transplant after donor organs are identified. For various reasons, the transplant was called off the first three times.

The fourth call was the one that would change his and Jeannie's lives. She stayed in an apartment near the hospital for several days after the transplant so that she could be with him as he recovered and learned about the new routine he would need to complete each day. The critical importance of taking the correct medications in a timely manner as prescribed each day is drilled into each new recipient.

A transplant recipient quickly learns the color, size, shape, and dosage of each pill. He knows what it is supposed to do and what the potential side effects are. He is also given new dietary and exercise restrictions to follow for at least the first few months.

Shortly after the surgery, the team of transplant physicians entered Steve's hospital room and surrounded his bedside. The doctors knew from previous interaction that Steve has a keen wit and splendid sense of humor. One of the doctors proceeded to inform Steve that, as a result of the surgery, he would now be a changed man. Somewhat concerned, Steve asked the doctor if he could be more specific as to how just how he would be a changed man. The doctor replied that Steve now has female parts. After a brief pause to ponder the new information, Steve responded, in a somewhat contemplative tone, that that would explain why he was tearing up so often since the surgery.

Steve's transplant was successful to the great joy of friends and family. He went back to work, after a brief recovery period, and continued to help support his family financially and to be there when they need him. He was looking forward to another transition in the not too distant future when he will begin a new life in retirement.

KAREN'S STORY

Many years after Ed's gift of life to me, I was working at the Bureau of Prisons central office in Washington, DC. I would often go for a brief exercise walk while at work during the lunch break. My office was just two blocks from the nation's capitol and the national mall. It is a beautiful and inspirational place to walk.

One day, after leaving the building for a drill, I noticed Karen, a friend and coworker sitting alone by the sidewalk. I had recently heard that she would be going on leave so that she could donate a kidney to a neighbor.

Karen had heard from one of her neighbors that Janet, another one of her neighbors, had recently started dialysis and was waiting for a transplant. Karen had signed up as an organ donor when she renewed her driver's license but did not know much about the process of living donation of organs so had never considered it.

Karen shared her story for a 2010 article in the *Washington Post* about the donation of organs by federal employees. She did not know Janet well but said, "When I heard of Janet's need, I never hesitated to say I would be tested. It was something I could do to help."

Karen had learned about a month earlier that her son and only child had been diagnosed with Hodgkin's disease. She had just returned from a visit to Oregon where she had taken her son to several chemo treatments. "As a mother, there is nothing worse than the news of cancer, and there is nothing you can do to personally make it go away," she said.

Karen did go through the entire process, and after a year of tests and waiting, transplant day arrived, and the two now celebrate their happy life day each year. It has now been more than ten years since transplant day, and though not all donors and recipients bond, Karen and Janet are good friends and have kept in touch over the years. They have celebrated the birth of grandbabies, Karen's 2007 wedding in Bermuda, and many other events together.

"I could never have imagined that part of donating," she said. (And by the way, her son is cancer-free.) This an amazing type of altruistic donation, and self-sacrifice is becoming more common as much advancement in transplantation have made it easier to match potential donors with recipients.

Living donors, like Karen, do have many questions to consider. What if something went wrong during surgery and assistance is needed for an extended period? What if she could no longer work and support herself? What if her remaining kidney someday became diseased? Would she regret that she had donated the other kidney? Would she be able to get health insurance in the future, if necessary, since she would only have one kidney?

For some, donation of an organ is just not possible, regardless of how willing they are to become an organ donor. And donors are not compensated for their gift beyond the costs they incur for testing and surgery. There are discussions within the industry to determine if that policy should change to allow for additional compensation to the donor. There are convincing arguments for both sides of the issue.

Paired kidney donation (PKD) has become more common in recent years. Paired exchange donation consists of two or more kidney donor/recipient pairs whose blood types are not compatible. The two recipients trade donors so that each recipient can receive a kidney with a compatible blood type. Once all donors and recipients have been tested, the kidney transplant surgeries can be scheduled to occur simultaneously.

DEBBIE'S STORY

Debbie is a friend, and Vandy buddy, that received a life-saving heart transplant at Vanderbilt a few short years ago. We did not know each other before discussing our common connection with Vanderbilt on Facebook. She is a beautiful woman with a remarkable spirit that is enjoying to the fullest her second chance at life. Our Vandy connection makes our friendship even more special, and I look forward to the day I can meet her in person and give her a hug.

Debbie was pacing the floor, unable to sleep, and afraid that she would not live through this night. She was in very bad shape and had only been home for a few hours after, yet another emergency trip and several days in the hospital at Vanderbilt. Her beloved dog of more than fourteen years had died while she was in the hospital adding to the trauma of the moment.

The silence of the night was suddenly broken when the phone rang. It was an official from Vanderbilt who told Debbie that a heart had become available for her. She woke her husband and told him it's time to go. Her bags were always packed and ready to go, and the car was kept full of gas. This night, however, they had to make a stop for gas at one of the few stations in town still open.

She gazed out the window of the car as they made the ninety-minute trip to Nashville noticing, under a full moon, every detail of the beautiful landscape. Though she had passed through the Land Between the Lakes many times, the scenery had never been more stirring.

She thought about the cherished hope that if she ever had the call for a transplant, she would walk into the hospital under her own strength when she arrived and not be carried in on a stretcher.

A Dobutamine drip was in her arm. At one point, her heart had stopped beating. The implanted cardioverter defibrillator (ICD) that was placed in her chest in a separate surgery shocked her heart and brought her back to consciousness. Doctors use the device to help treat irregular heartbeats. An ICD uses electrical pulses or shocks to help control life-threatening arrhythmias, especially those that can cause sudden cardiac arrest (SCA). Her doctors at Vanderbilt had helped keep her alive for more than four years.

She entered the emergency room at about 2:30 in the morning. The young man at the desk told her to stop and asked how he could help her. The maintenance men were busy buffing the floors, and it was difficult for them to hear one another speak over roar of the machines. Out of breath, she hollered at him as best she could, "I'm here to get a heart transplant." He tells her that she must go to the fifth floor but, for some reason, did not offer her a wheelchair.

Debbie meandered through the long hallways trying to get to the elevator but must make a detour around a roped off area where another maintenance man is replacing tile on the floor and will not let her pass. She finally reached the fifth floor still unsure if she will make it when she realized she has gone the wrong way down the corridor. It seemed to take forever to get to the transplant surgery center on the other end of Vanderbilt, but she did. Fear now replaced the determination she had to make it this far.

In Debbie's situation, friends and family did not live close enough to offer assistance or provide care. Her father had died in 1999 after a fall from a deer stand. Her mother lived in San Diego, where Debbie had grown up, but had recently suffered a heart attack and was unable to travel. Her three brothers each lived in different states and had families of their own. She endured the four and a half years since being diagnosed with heart disease mostly alone with the exception of her husband.

Debbie had accomplished her goal of walking into the hospital, and it was a true blessing to her. This was her standout moment. She now fondly remembers the funny part. It was the time she walked through the hospital late at night and all alone to receive a heart transplant. She reminded us that she was not alone. God was walking with her. She was reminded of this again by the three doves on the window sill. The three doves she saw as she walked into her hospital room for her first surgery a few years earlier.

Debbie's symptoms began on her fortieth birthday. She was retaining fluid and short of breath. Visits to several doctors and attempts to control the symptoms were unsuccessful until a doctor in her hometown of Murray, Kentucky, diagnosed her with heart failure. He told her that she should travel to Vanderbilt University Medical Center as soon as possible. Not good timing for a mother of three boys, but is there ever good timing for anyone?

Debbie spent the next thirty-two days in the Cardiac Intensive Care Unit (CICU) where her condition rapidly deteriorated. Two large bottles of fluid were drained from her body, but fluid quickly returned. She was taken to surgery where six more bottles of fluid were drained. Debbie is a fighter, and she survived the ordeal for the time being. Pneumonia and blood clots were just a few of the issues that developed over the next few weeks.

As the possibility of a heart transplant drew closer, representatives with her health insurance company informed her that the insurance company would not pay for her transplant if it was performed at Vanderbilt instead of another hospital that they had designated. She was very satisfied with the treatment that she had received at Vanderbilt and had made friends with many of the doctors, nurses, and staff. She did not want to start the process over at another hospital. The problems with the insurance company were eventually resolved with assistance from the head of the Vanderbilt transplant team and several other people.

She was now eligible to be placed on the transplant waiting list but suffered another setback when an eligibility review determined that she was ineligible for transplant because of pulmonary hypertension. The emotional roller-coaster ride continued when her doctor told her that the hypertension had stabilized and she could proceed with the listing.

Her health continued to deteriorate, and on one occasion, her heart stopped beating. Although she did recover, nagging doubts and fear continued. Would she live long enough to receive a transplant? After one dry run, on January 9, 2008, she received the call that would change her life.

Debbie has made many friends at Vanderbilt and enjoys the opportunity to visit with them when she returns for follow-up visits. Her new heart has allowed her to once again enjoy an active lifestyle. She knows all too well how fragile life is and never takes for granted the gift she has received.

ORGAN DONATION IS NOT AN EASY DECISION

While some friends have made the decision to donate or to receive a transplant, other friends have had to make the terrible decision of whether to donate organs of a family member who has tragically died. This is a situation that no one ever wants a family to encounter. At what is probably the worst moments of their lives they must quickly and decisively determine whether their loved one should become a donor.

Many have died waiting for a life-saving transplant, and thousands more are on the waiting list today. I was one of the fortunate ones who received a life-saving organ transplant. Ed was almost a perfect match.

The heroes, of course are the donors, are living and deceased who have given the gift of life. The recipients inherit a responsibility to do what they can to maintain the gift, including a lifetime of immunosuppressant medications, which often have unwanted side effects. Some of the side effects may develop quickly, others may develop over time.

WHAT HAPPENS AFTER A TRANSPLANT

Certainly, not all transplants are successful in the short term, and longevity is not guaranteed. While many transplant patients get back to a normal life posttransplant, others struggle with episodes of rejection, affordability of medications, insurance problems, and other illnesses that may negatively impact the grafted organ. Families often struggle along with the patient through years of uncertainty.

Those without adequate finances and insurance may be forced to limit or stop taking the medication necessary to maintain the transplant. Medicare, for those who qualify, may help pay for some expenses, but it does not cover all expenses, and it usually expires two years after the transplant, leaving those without insurance or financial wealth with heartbreaking decisions.

For those who suffer from life-altering illness, the endless doctor visits and painful, humiliating treatments are only part of the story. Life becomes immediate and the future less certain. One's freedom to move may be severely restricted. Routine travel for pleasure or business can be extremely limited.

A transplant patient may have strict dietary limits on food and beverage consumption. Social interaction may be reduced, and friendships are often tested. Finances and questions about health insurance may be constant worries. Loneliness and an uncertain future add to the worries. Faith is called upon to prove its worth as never before.

It seemed we don't think about serious illness until it happens to us or a loved one. Especially as young people, we tend to think and hope that it will never happen to us. But the chances are that each of us may someday face the challenge of dealing with and hopefully conquering a life altering disease. From multiple sclerosis to cancer, diabetes, heart, lung, or other organ disease, to aids or the many other forms of illness, each must face the challenges and make the decisions, hopefully with the help and assistance of loved ones.

PHOTOS

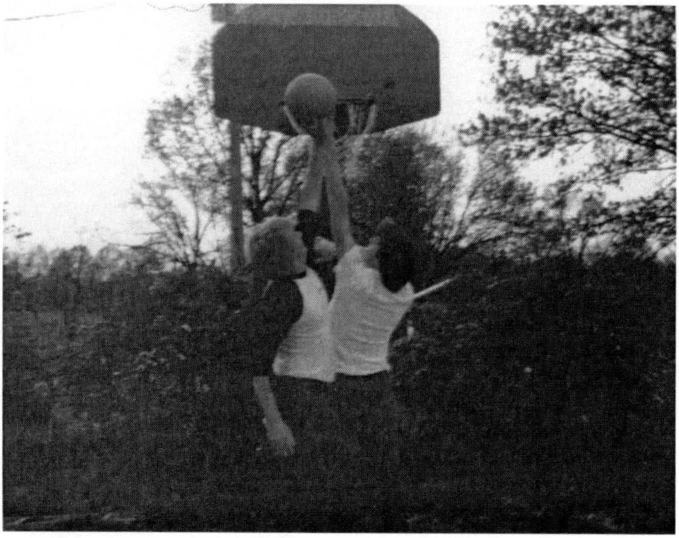

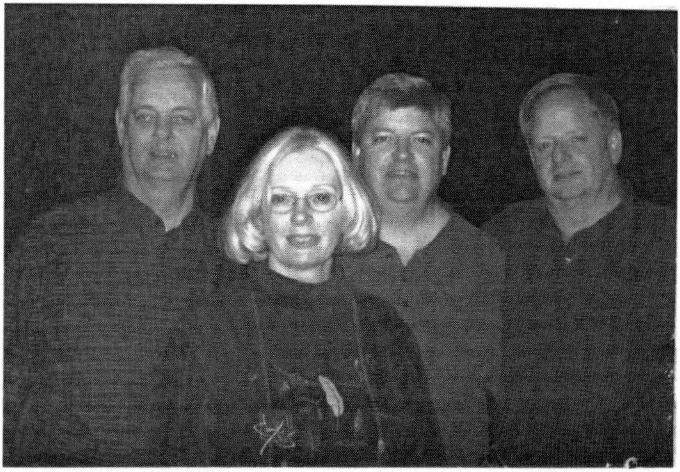

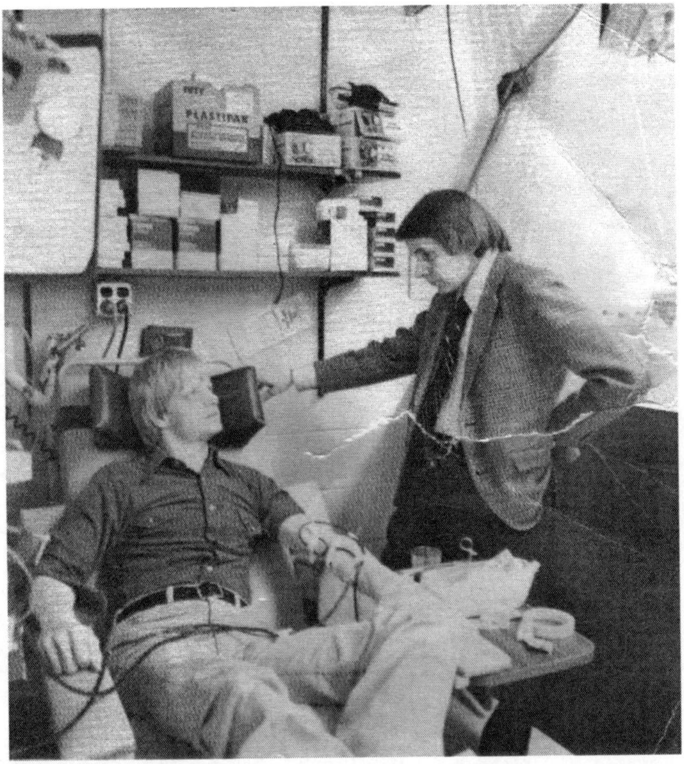
PLASTIPAK

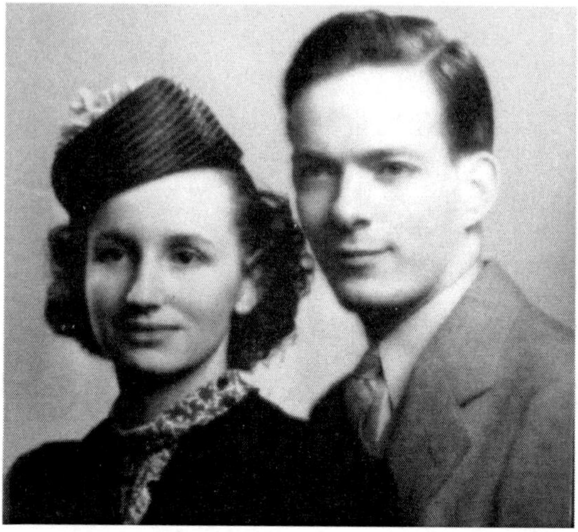

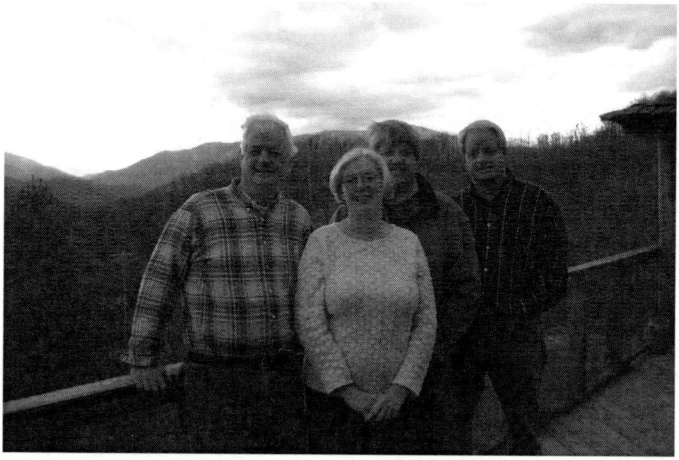